Choices

Inspiring Stories of Healing Through Alternative and Holistic Health Care

19 Authors Sharing Real Stories of

Hope and Healing

Cherri Gregori-Pedrioli

Choices Book Series

www.ChoicesBookSeries.com

Choices
Inspiring Stories of Healing Through Alternative and Holistic Health Care
Copyright © 2019 by Holistic Choices Publishing

Holistic Choices Publishing

For Information address:

Holistic Choices Publishing
609 Jean Marie Drive
Santa Rosa, CA 95403

In conjunction with
GWYW Publishing
1230 Crescent Dr.
Glendale, CA 91205

Dedication

I dedicate this book to two of the most amazing and important women in my life; my grandmother Minnie (Gregori) Chavez and my mother Barbara Jean (Roberts) Gregori.

I know in my heart, that had you both explored your Choices, the outcome may have been very different.

Because of the events of your life, and the journey I walked with you, I have the strength, the courage, and the knowledge to spread the word about Choices.

"In the end that was the choice you made, and it doesn't matter how hard it was to make it. It matters that you did."
— Cassandra Clare, City of Glass

Table of Contents

Foreword

by Susan Sheppard

It was 1965 in a highly reputable Illinois teaching hospital, prior to Coronary Care Units. It was well known, at that time, that only men over the age of 50 experienced Heart attacks, so they were treated with six weeks of absolute bedrest in hospital without any monitoring.

A 27-year-old young man walked up to the Emergency window and told me he was having chest pain. I started to send him to the waiting room until we had a bed in a minor room for colds. I felt a psychic jab in my shoulder and changed my mind. I escorted him to our newly designated cardiac room and asked him to undress so I could take an EKG. When I returned to the room, his heart had stopped. I called for help and started CPR. We saved his life. The lesson for me was "pay attention to what your body is communicating". It will save you and your patients' lives. This was my first recognized experience of intuition, and believe me, I paid attention for the next 39 years of Emergency nursing. I believe thousands of my patients were saved by my intuition jabs. It led me to study Extra Sensory Perception, Intuition, Neuro Linguistic Programming, Hypnosis, EFT, and several other modalities of other than conscious communication and healing.

My publishing company arose from frustration with traditional and hybrid publishing houses who required my writing, my marketing, and my publicity for them to keep the profits. My initial intention was to publish more than 20 of my own books about life, business, and relationship coaching.

Then I participated in about three compilation books where I wrote a part of my story for each of them.

What occurred each time was a release of energy and pent up emotions that I had stored for many years. That was an interesting experience. When Sue Brooke, (*Choices Book Series* producer and co-publisher), suggested we publish a compilation book, *Discover your Identity*. I said why not? It seemed like a great idea, and recognizing the entrepreneurial brain that I have, it was just another venture. What occurred, because many of the authors were first time authors and didn't know how to go about writing a story, was my first experience coaching a new writer to share their truth. It was definitely a learning experience for all of us, and many of the writer's had amazing emotional breakthroughs.

The next book that we published, *Discover your Inspiration*, was an even better experience of authors having personal development breakthrough experiences that were unpredictable. Even more of the authors were first timers and required more and more coaching. I started to understand that the process of writing a personal story was an avenue of personal growth that led each individual to a peak moment that allowed them to release the emotions of fear, anger, hurt, shame, guilt and sadness that they had stored for many years.

The biggest revelation for me occurred when Sue and I attended a retreat for Bridge leaders. Bridges is a non-profit organization that assists lay people in a religious community to reach out to others and share their faith and then develop their own non-profit organization devoted to many and different causes. We supported these Bridge leaders to write their own stories that led them to their mission. These people had no experience of writing, and many had severe anxieties about revealing their private thoughts and feelings regarding their personal tragedies, crises, and often criminal incidents that led them to their individual mission. I became the conduit to help them understand that revealing these, often embarrassing, dangerous, and violent incidents would release their pent-up emotions and fears that they had harbored for many years. Some of these, now religious leaders, were prior criminals, rape victims, molested children, unwed mothers, drug abusers, and drunks. The experience of writing down their story and sharing it, allowed them to release their inhibitions, heal their emotional trauma, and grow as a human being.

Which leads us to this book, *Choices*. It has been my honor to support each of the authors in this book to reveal some of their most guarded secrets, to share with the world the incidents that led each of them to their holistic path. The stories are bold, direct and often traumatic, which only accentuates the authenticity of these dedicated professionals. Each author underwent a profound personal transformation as they revealed and wrote their chapter. It is a privilege to have been of assistance in their personal growth.

Susan Sheppard is the CEO of Getting What You Want, Inc., a Life Coaching organization that specializes in helping singles grow their self-esteem and expand their perception of who is available for relationship with them. She is an author, a speaker, a publisher and a retired Emergency Services RN. **www.GettingWhatYouWant.com**

Acknowledgements

There are so many to thank for the opportunity in writing and publishing the first book in the Choices Book Series.

First off, a huge thank you to Sue Brooke for seeing the vision and having the faith and trust in me in bringing my story to light. Sue said we all have a story and who knew that in writing just one chapter would be so healing. Thanks for the countless hours that you have spent on this project. Now I am a Night Owl.

Susan Sheppard for all the time you spent with helping the authors including me in guiding us to dig deep.

Thank you to my parents William and Jeanie Gregori for teaching me life's lessons and how hard work pays off and to never give up.

Thank you to my grandmother Minnie Gregori Chavez for always believing in me and encouraging me to follow my dreams.

Thank you to all of the contributing authors in the first book by sharing your story of Healing in Alternative and Holistic Healthcare. Diana Borges, thanks for all the Heart talks, Deborah Myers, thanks for the lessons on self-care, Karen and Robert Wagner, thanks for always being there with positive support, Elizabeth Smith for all your help in putting our system together, Patrice Fistor-Jaehnig for being a mentor, office partner and friend, Janet Caliri for the tools that you taught me to be able to look at my house again, and to my new friends and fellow authors Kari Joly' Estill, Janet Briscoe-Smith, Susan Maddux, June Boertee, Addie Spahr Kim, Christi Corradi, Kristi Oen, Simon Emsley, Juliet Carrillo, Maghen Ward, Angela Legh, I love each and every one of you and appreciate your patience in this journey together.

Thanks to my husband Duane for putting up with my crazy hours and schedules and letting me be me, even though you don't get what I do, you have always been there for me. You are the hardest working man I know; we have had our fair shares of downs in life, but we survived it all. Thank you for everything. I Love You

Thanks to my kids John Jones and Jeanie Lombardi for allowing me to be your mom which has taught me so many valuable life's lessons. I truly believe we fight for survival and strength for our children and I wanted to be here for the two of you and be the mom that you were proud of. I Love You

Thanks to my Custom Plumbing office staff for holding down the fort; Nanci Stewart, Ed Anderson and Craig Wagner, without you guys I would not of had the time that was needed for this project.

Thanks to all my family and friends for all the love and support.

Cherri Gregori-Pedrioli

Introduction

by Cherri Gregori-Pedrioli

How important is your life?

My whole life, as long as I can remember, I wanted to help everyone that I loved. It makes me sad when I see people I love and care about going down the wrong path. There are so many Choices out there that can help people.

As a Child, a Daughter, a Mother, a Sibling, a Friend, a Spouse, an Employee, and an Employer, I have watched the destruction of disease, mental illness, addiction and abuse. All of life's challenges that I either participated in or observed, were very valuable lessons that led me to explore the nuances of Choices.

Most people struggle with change. It intimidates them, it challenges them, it stops them. WHY? The answer to this paralyzing predicament is they want to explore their Choices but are unsure of where to start.

Why do we struggle so much with Choices? Maybe it is overwhelming, maybe we don't have enough information, maybe we don't know how to begin exploring our Choices.

Life, for many, has not always been about Choice. We should have Choices in everything we do in life; decisions about education, relationships, where we live, what we eat, what we wear, and of course, our health care. We were not born depressed, suicidal, addicted to pharmaceuticals, drugs or alcohol, and we were not born to bully or be bullied. For example, in regard to mental illness, big pharma is supporting the self-destruction of people every day. I have witnessed firsthand, many experiencing the cycle of depression and anxiety by prescribed pill after pill after pill with the result being drug dependence, progressing to self-medication, then addiction, and often street drugs to satisfy their cravings.

When it comes to our health care, Fear takes away our Freedom of Choice.

Growing up, I wasn't given the Choice about my health care, all I knew was to trust what I was told, and we learned from watching others. If I had listened to my doctors many years ago, my life would be very different, and I would not have my children or grandchildren. Today, it is about educating our community around Choices in Alternative and Holistic Health Care. Frequently, modern medicine treats symptoms without searching for the core issues. Many accepted treatments are just Band-Aids. You are the owner of your body; therefore, you really need to do your own research about what is happening in the various systems of your body. The focus of alternative and holistic health care includes exploring the root issues of your symptoms. Choices is about bridging the gap and introducing Alternative and Holistic Health Care, with the intention of expanding Western Medicine, not replacing it.

When you're sick and tired of being sick and tired, you will decide to take the next step of exploring your Choices. You must remember that there is no easy fix to any situation; it takes work, determination, drive, but most importantly you have to want to be better.

So, you explored some choices when it comes to your health, now what? Who do you see? What is the best approach? Who do you trust? What is best for you?

This first issue of *Choices* will offer you some unique, interesting, effective alternatives to assist you with your research.

Holistic Choices Inc. and Choices Books Series are a steppingstone for many. The stories in this book are real stories and real life-changing events, from just a small handful of authors who have experienced life changing events all because they explored their Choices.

Choices are everywhere, so do yourself a favor, do the research and explore those Choices.

Chapter 1

The Beautiful Scar

by Elizabeth Beaty-Smith

"Only when it is dark can you see the stars"

I like to run my fingers over the scar and admire the symmetrical set of dots that run along my wrist that once stitched my artery back together. It is a reminder of the power in my choices, and that sometimes even the wrong choices, can bring us to the right places.

I made a choice to take a razor blade from my grandmother's old toiletry box. I sat in my green-tiled bathroom on the wicker laundry hamper and ran the blade along my wrist deep enough to feel exactly the release I had needed.

The events that led to my suicide attempt was a result of chronic trauma. I did not have the tools to help me self-regulate or cope with the physical and emotional symptoms I was experiencing, so I trusted a medical team to "cure" me.

For about 5 months, my care consisted of taking 18 pills a day, attending 15 hours a week of intensive counseling, 3 different doctors and 2 therapists. How could I even consider taking my life with all that medical intervention? How does one get to that state of mind that they can do something like that; to be selfish enough to leave behind a child, family, friends, or job?

When I was 20, I got a job at a hospital. I was a fast and eager learner. I was trained in 10 different departments and would often bounce around, helping each. The hospital was struggling, with budget cuts so severe it was dangerous for staff and patients. For example, a department that would operate with 25 employees was now being forced to operate with 3. Employees were forced to work overtime under hostile working conditions created by management. I suppose you could say I blew the whistle and made management accountable for the choices they were making. I was told to shut my mouth "or else." Although I stand by the choices I made, I can admit that I took on too much, and made the issues my own. I had joined several committees, trying to boost morale hospital wide and be sure employees felt appreciated and heard. It began to consume me, literally.

My health began to suffer, and it started to manifest physically and emotionally. I began bleeding vaginally, suffered from chronic migraines, heart palpitations, insomnia, short term memory loss, obsessive thoughts, anger, anxiety attacks, nightmares, high blood pressure, and a plethora of other symptoms. I went to my primary care doctor and he encouraged me to take pills. I was hesitant and declined, at least at first. When I had asked for something holistic, he told me that this is western medicine and to go for a run. Finally, I was told if I did not take the pills, I could no longer be seen. Fearful and feeling cornered, I agreed, and within a few weeks I went from a couple of low dose prescriptions, to 9 different prescriptions, taking 18 pills a day. I now felt like a zombie, still experiencing the same symptoms and the side effects of the medication, unable to care for myself, or my young son. I was doing everything the medical team told me, yet I felt worse. I had begun having anxiety attacks so intense that I could no longer drive and was then dependent on others to drive me.

I got lost in the medical system and had to stop some of this madness. I told the doctors and therapists that I was beginning to feel like I wanted to harm myself and/or others. It felt like they didn't hear me. Not getting the help I so desperately needed, I admitted myself into a mental health facility for a week, hoping for answers. They ran a series of tests, more counseling, and added a pill that I had a terrible reaction to, that caused me to scratch my arms up with my nail-bitten hands so badly that both forearms were bandaged for weeks. My meds continued to be increased while in their care, almost capping out at the highest dosages. Finally, I was given a diagnosis of PTSD. That same day I was asked if I wanted to kill myself still, I said yes, and they said, sorry, there is nothing more we can do, because I was not a veteran experiencing PTSD, and they sent me home.

Once I got home, I begged the medical team to wean me off the pills. They did not think it was a good idea, and told me, "No".

I sat in my backyard with a razor blade. It started out as light scratches that started to get deeper. I felt out of control. I was desperate to not feel the surge of electricity I had inside, and the blade was able to provide a release. My survival instincts kicked in and drove me to use social media to post that I really needed help. Someone noticed and came to me. By the time they arrived, my judgement was severely impaired, and I ran to my bathroom. Laughing madly, I dug the blade in as deep as I could. I couldn't even process what I had done, I had a towel over my wrist and would pull it back to just watch the blood rush out of my body, which covered the entire bathroom floor. As the paramedics put me on a gurney, I lost consciousness before I got to the ambulance. I was given stitches and blood transfusions in the emergency room and was transported to mental health where they did not 5150 me. They released me to my mother's care. The next day, I woke up in my mom's bed feeling clarity-determined to heal myself. I googled 'Holistic Retreats' and came across one an hour away. I was able to spend 2 days there, in nature; journaling, meditating, and had visions of healing others with my experience.

I decided to stop the pills, cold turkey. I was not prepared for the withdrawal symptoms, which were almost unbearable. I felt like the medical team did not support me, as I was no longer taking their pills. Luckily, I had a supportive community, friends, and family that stood by my side.

I was encouraged to try Yoga, by a friend. It was intimidating, however, I was determined to heal, so I attended a class at the gym. Even with the basketballs banging on the wall, I knew this was going to change my life forever. It was a safe space to feel my emotions, to move in a way that released the tension and the pain that my weak body felt. I was able to breathe into the spaces that had lacked oxygen from holding my breath. I craved more. I was invited to attend 'Wanderlust', a beautiful festival full of music, art, nature, Yoga, meditation, and healthy food. I spent most of the time alone; feeling so enlightened, surrounded by this new whole world I was exposed to.

While in the mental health facility, and at 'Wanderlust', I was exposed to art and music therapy. It was a space where I could express myself; feeling freedom that came from being submerged in colors, brush strokes, feeling textures with my hands, hearing emotion in the music, feeling the bass that sang to my soul, it made me feel alive. I felt compelled to share with others who needed to feel a relief from the pain, so I collaborated with Mental Health to offer suicide support groups. I wanted to continue a path that would expose people to all the new things I was learning, so they would know they had choices in their healing journey.

I made the choice to quit my job shortly after my suicide attempt, as I knew I had found my mission: To share the tools I had learned about to prevent suicide and to heal. I have devoted my work to children and families, and bringing the tools of self-regulation, breathing, self-soothing techniques, art, movement, and resiliency, into schools, the community, and the home.

I stand in my power to know that I have choices, and I am empowered to be my own advocate for health. I chose to be authentically me, embracing my trauma, loving myself for who I am. Even if I am not fully recovered, I choose to live my life with an open mind, surrounding myself with people and environments that inspire and educate me, as I continue grow.

Some do not understand why I make myself vulnerable and pour my heart out for the world to see my biggest flaw. I am proud to be alive. To run my fingers over this enormous beautiful scar that has allowed me to live bigger than I ever could have imagined.

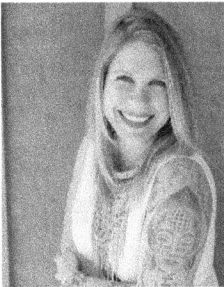

Elizabeth Beaty-Smith is an authentic creator, entrepreneur, inspirational public speaker, has a passion for community, and is a Soroptimist. She moved to Sebastopol, CA, with her family, to flourish her business and to soak up all the culture and good vibes.

Elizabeth is a Registered Yoga instructor and a Registered Children's Yoga instructor certified in 6 different modalities of Yoga. She was a trainer for an Internationally recognized children's yoga program. She holds certifications in Cognitive Behavior Therapy, Child Psychology, Strengthening Families™ Protective Factors Framework, Suicide Prevention, Therapeutic Art, and Personal Training. Elizabeth is the founder of Project Whole Child, which specializes in Early Childhood Education and school age children. The program focuses on the child's Village, Health and Nutrition, Emotional Wellbeing, and Physical Wellbeing. She believes they are just as important as ABCs and 123s.

The Arts and Yoga became significant tools for healing her PTSD and her suicide attempt in 2012. Elizabeth has begun the process of starting a non-profit called Project H;ART. The semi-colon comes from the movement, Project Semicolon. The mission is to educate and inspire others to use alternative methods of healing suicide trauma such as music, art, and movement. Having seen the healing power of the human body in her own experiences, she hopes others can find an outlet that can help them to heal and grow. Elizabeth wants to help break down the walls of stigma surrounding suicide and create a world where social prescribing is used universally.

www.ProjectWholeChild.com

Chapter 2
Crossing the Threshold to Possibilities by
Diana Borges

*"Reconnect. Release. Rejoice. Experiencing Is
Believing" ~Diana Borges*

The tuning forks glided up his chest and settled on the area his body
had signaled. The ends of the weighted forks pulsed into the heart
area, waves knocking at its protective layer before traveling down
his torso. Spencer's forehead scrunched, drawing his eyebrows
closer. His words echoed in my head; wife, kids, work, not going
well. Shut down, not present.

The areas near his temples welcomed the vibrating forks. Saying
hello, first to the busy monkey brain, then modulating the energy a
little more with each additional strike. His lips parted, releasing a
slow sigh, and his body sagged closer to the table.

My hands returned the forks to his heart, the key for him to know his
truth and reconnect to his own power. The forks struck the leg pad
and again returned to his area of most resistance. Liquid formed near
the corner of one eyelid and our hearts synced. "Take a deep breath,"
I advised. "That's it. Let whatever is coming up process so it can be
released."

The vibrations drained from the forks into his body, deeper and
deeper, filling the void within his chest. If he only knew that the
illusional layer protecting his heart not only kept him from having
deeper love for himself and his family, but also from experiencing
life's possibilities.

"How are you doing?" I inquired.

Bleak eyes drifted in my direction, and his shoulders shrugged. The clash between moving forward and staying in his comfort zone now playing on his consciousness.

"We are going to start the Heart Access journey now," I said, my back resting against the webbed desk chair. "But first, I want to explain something. We are here in this life to learn, evolve, love, and to experience all of life-even the things we interpret as bad. Many are learning opportunities for us to grow." A grave look appeared up at me. "There is usually a bigger picture unfolding for us that we may not be aware of. Reconnecting to your heart and soul can bring about wondrous things. Believe in yourself more." Our eyes penetrated each other.

I continued. "Okay, let's begin. I want you to start by feeling your physical heart within your chest." My fingertips rested on his left forearm, like those on piano keys, waiting to conduct a transformational melody. "We are going to journey to a place beyond your physical heart...Good. I invite you to open the door to your heart and step inside. Know this is a safe place, because it is your own heart."

Working together, more doors and windows within his heart opened, clearing passages that held hindering energies from this life and beyond. Fear, pain, guilt, and even worthlessness flowed out on the exhaled air and down his body to Earth. Emotions, that had only been known to his subconscious, releasing more and more.

My teeth bit my upper lip. "Divine guides help, please." My head tilted back, and a sinking sensation traveled down my spine. "Spencer," I began, "I invite you to set the intent to release the old programs…those stories on your cellular and subconscious levels that do not serve your highest good. Allow energies that are holding you back to be released. You don't even need to know the details.

They will arise if necessary." My shoulders lowered, and a smirk formed on my face.

Layers floated off tiny cells scattered throughout his body. Cells energetically freed from dragging around illusions that held him back. "I invite you to now download from the divine that which is for your highest good. Allow this new information to reside on your cells, your subconscious, and anywhere else that is appropriate for your highest good, your evolutionary path, and your purpose here."

My eyes squinted, attempting to fine tune the blurred internal vision. The video in my head focused, and an elated feeling enveloped me. A boy chasing a beagle puppy in circles played on my eyelid projector screen. High pitched yelps and laughter filled the air around them. Joy and excitement present in their collective energy field. A window suddenly burst open, and a man's voice bellowed out. The boy's feet planted on the grass like the taproot of a White Oak tree. The child scooped up the panting puppy and shuffled into the house. The door slamming as they crossed the threshold.

My fingertips pressed slightly on Spencer's skin. "I invite you to go back to a time in your childhood. To the place where your little boy self needs our attention." The energy field surrounding us formed an energetic tunnel, and a towering man peered into the eyes of his eight-year-old self.

"I want you to take the boy's hand. Tell him he is safe. Tell him we are here to help him." My eyes gazed at the heavenly bamboo swaying outside the window. "Ask him what he needs from us, and how we can help him."

Spencer's arm twitched beneath my fingers. "Tell him he is loved. Tell him he is worthy just how he is...No matter what anyone says."

Spencer's breathing quickened, forcing the lump in his throat to dissolve. Compassion for the child's situation, and forgiveness for himself, blossomed within.

"It is time to bring those energies back to the present," I announced. "Incorporate the energies into who you are now, they have been harmonized. He is part of you, and always has been."

Our collective energy field expanded, filling the room first, then extending beyond the walls. "I invite your soul to be present, that energetic part of you. Feel who you truly are, beyond the physical constraints. Know that you have the ability to self-heal and that all the answers you seek are within you. I invite you to have unconditional love, compassion, and patience for yourself. Because it starts with each and every one of us." I connected his heart to Earth's heart, introducing him to grounded awareness. "It is only after we take care of ourselves will these emotions genuinely overflow to others, life, and our physical world."

His motionless body remained on the table as the clock ticked away. Glazed eyes surveyed his palms, bouncing from one to the other.

"Um, how are you?" I said, testing the waters. Deer in headlight eyes glanced in my direction. "I don't know," a distraught voice responded. "My hands, my palms...I can't shut them off. It feels like energy is flowing off of them. I don't know what to do."

My left hand attempted to conceal a chuckle. "I am sorry for laughing. But that is a good thing. Here, let me help you." Energy from my palms pulsed into his, the right one first then the left, quickening with each cycle. I visualized the energy flowing back into his hands, then set the intent for his palms to seal off, so that he could consciously decide when to send energy. "How does that feel?" I asked, scanning his face.

He nodded. "Better. What happened?"

My right hand clutched my chest. "You reconnected to your heart and soul, that energetic part of you. That is where our power is. Our truth." A sigh expelled from my lips. "There are many things that happen over our lifetime that disempower us. Things we are told. Other people's stories we believe, and emotions we suppress. But you now have a different understanding of the things that happened in your life."

"It will take some time to completely process what you experienced." My shoulders shrugged and head tilted. "Allow yourself to process in whatever way you need. Are we still on for another session next week?" I asked, as he gave me a hug.

"Definitely, even more after today," his hand reached for the doorknob.

Spencer and I have worked together eight times within the past year, and we plan to take his transformation even further. Because of his broadened perceptions of who he is and his willingness to heal, he has shifted his internal and external worlds. His relationships with his wife, children, and himself have improved, and the product he was attempting to design at the beginning is now in the testing stage. He once told me that the tuning forks bring him in touch with his body, the guided journey into his heart and brain takes him into his subconscious, and expansion of his energy allows him to see the collective energy field.

When I am asked to describe my perfect client, I fondly recall Spencer, the gentle soul who trusted enough to rediscover his own true nature.

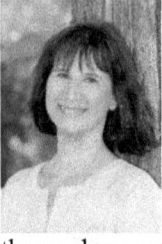

Diana Borges releases blockages and broadens perceptions so you can live a healthy and successful life. She empowers others with their innate knowledge and strength, allowing for self-healing, personal growth and joy. With Diana's guidance, her clients have had profound transformations by removing limiting beliefs, believing in themselves more, and seeing beyond the day to day physical world. Diana is a life coach, energy healer, speaker and author who draws on her own life experiences, education, channeling skills, and ability to move energy. She is a certified Life Purpose Coach, a certified HeartMath Institute Add Heart Facilitator, a certified tuning forks practitioner under The Biofield Tuning Institute, Reiki Master, Former Co-President of the Santa Rosa Holistic Chamber of Commerce and one of the chapter's founding members.

Diana is the creator of Heart Access, a unique energetic modality. She is also the founder of Whole Earth Hub, which offers a Heart Talk Series, Earth Talk Series and earthly meditations. Diana has a B.S. degree in Geology from the University of California, Davis, California. She has been a Registered Geologist in the State of California since 1994, primarily assisting in the physical healing of Earth by investigating and remediating contamination. She was President, and Partner of a successful environmental consulting firm for about 8 years. Prior to that, she was the Environmental Division Manager for a separate consulting firm for 13 years.

www.BorgesExperience.com

Chapter 3
The Little Girl and the Medicine Man
by Cherri Gregori-Pedrioli

"May your choices reflect your hopes, not your fears." ~Nelson Mandela

It all started on the playground at Oak Grove Elementary school when I was 10 years old. I was sitting with a group of my little friends, telling stories. I can't quite remember how it all transpired, or what we were talking about, but what I do remember is telling the kids that I could Heal them, just like my Indian medicine man grandfather. My teacher told me that I needed to stop telling those stories because I was scaring the other kids. She even called my parents and I got in trouble for my story telling. Was this the wild imagination of a child, or the child who knew that we all carry the innate ability to heal others?

As you continue to read my story you will wonder, how on earth did I evolve to this person I am today and why I feel so strong and passionate that we all need to explore our Choices!

When I was 13, some kids started a rumor about me having sex, which of course was not true. They called me a slut, and other hurtful, ugly names. I was traumatized, hurt, and embarrassed. I just wanted to escape. Unsure of where to turn for help, my escape was the introduction to pills and alcohol to help me forget. I existed in a fog, just to not feel the pain. Staying numb kept the hurt away, until it came to that point where I just could not take it anymore, I wanted to end my life, so I took a handful of different pills and drank them down with vodka. I ended up in the hospital where they actually prescribed me even more pills. I hated my situation, and I knew I had to do something different, but what?

Still struggling with the trauma from my junior high years, I continued, occasionally, to stay numb with pills and alcohol. This is when life took another toll on me. In my junior year of high school, a friend and I were at a high school game and decided to walk to town. On the way back, two guys asked us if we wanted a ride, and we accepted. We thought it was very nice of them and they seemed harmless. They offered us a drink, which we accepted, not knowing the drinks were drugged until we woke up on the side of the road, altered and sexually violated...completely unaware of what had happened to us. The next day we reported the incident to the police, but their investigation was fruitless. After months into the investigation the charges were dropped. So, for me, I took another step towards emotional bankruptcy. I graduated to smoking pot more regularly, along with other mind-altering substances to numb the pain of the rape. It was so much easier to stay numb and just stay busy, avoiding all feelings.

At one point I decided that I needed to make a change in my life, so I thought by following in my Grandmother's path of caretaking and healing, it just may help me with my own struggles. I became a Certified Nurse's Aide and worked in a Convalescent home. I watched the elderly patients become lethargic and continue to decline, while the medical professionals fed them more and more drugs. I began to really question Western medicine.

Even though I continued to follow the traditional Western Medical path, there was doubt in my mind, and I was suspicious of their intentions and results.

After the birth of my son at age 18, I suffered from excruciating pain in my right ovary. My doctor told me I had to have a total hysterectomy, and removing my ovaries was the only solution or I would die from the toxins that were in my body. I refused to believe that this was true. The glimmer of hope that non-traditional, holistic, shamanic, or whatever alternate healing powers existed, gave me the strength to ignore his prognosis. Validation of my new beliefs occurred when I gave birth to my second child, a daughter.

In 1996 I lost one of the most amazing women in my life...my grandmother. She was diagnosed with Lung Cancer; the tumor was the size of a dime. Her doctors convinced her to get in a clinical trial, as they felt it was her only hope of survival. She was diagnosed in May, treatments started at the end of June, and she passed away July 9th. Cause of Death: Suffocation. Her doctors never collaborated with one another, she should have never been put in the trial, she had emphysema and COPD. My faith in Western Medicine was now really being questioned.

So, once again, I went on another downward spiral. Needing to stay numb, I started taking pills again and, of course, drinking. I was at a point in my life where I just existed. Taking pills were now part of my normal because while I was growing up, Western medical doctors were all about pills and surgery. Everyone was taking some kind of pill...it seems funny now, but when we were kids, they told us to stay away from them because they would hurt us.

Although my faith in alternative healing was growing stronger, the physical pain intensified and I surrendered to pain relief once again, with prescriptions and street drugs. I continued on that path because that is what I knew.

I remember, around 2005, after a night of partying, I thought I was dying. Fortunately, it turned out to be the side effects from the pills and drugs I was taking. I needed to get my life back...I was tired of just existing in a numb world. I told my husband that I was done. No more drugs of any kind, no pills, no nothing.

My journey took me to a Shaman, a Medicine Man... remember the little girl and the medicine man? He asked me to lie down and put a cloth over my eyes. I smelled sage burning and heard people chanting. Soon he stopped and told me that he had found the problem, to lay still, and that it would hurt just for a moment. I felt a sharp pain in my right ovary, and I saw, in my mind's eye, something crystalize, then travel down my leg, and exit through my feet! I was in shock...the pain was gone!

Several months later, I woke up with a 103-degree fever, a horrible pain in my side and back, and peeing blood. A friend told me to call my doctor right away, because it was probably a bladder or kidney infection. I chose to call the Shaman instead. While on the phone, he told me to lay still while he took a look at what was going on. Once again, he told me it would only hurt for a moment. Five minutes later, the pain and fever were gone! He told me that he removed a kidney stone. Again, I was in shock! How could this happen? He was 850 miles away!

My Shamanic Journey was the catalyst that would lead me to seek out other Choices in Alternative and Holistic Health Care.

Over the years I continued to struggle with other health issues and continued to explore my Choices, because it was time to live life on my terms. As I continued down my path of exploration, a friend recommended that I have a Reconnective Healing® session, and from that day forward my life was changed.

I originally went to the session for a physical healing, but what I received was an awakening that lead me on a mission to educate my family, friends and my community that they too have Choices that should be explored before making life changing decisions.

Some of my own healing experiences were from spiritual awareness to physical healings such as; a broken finger that healed by the next day, a mass in my breast disappeared, a neck injury healed back to normal, and torn chest cartilage healed in front of an audience at the training seminar I was attending, where I was to become a Reconnective Healing® practitioner.

I opened my practice after a friend of mine was diagnosed with Stage 4 Multiple Myeloma and given no more than 2 years to live. She tried everything from Western Medicine to Holistic Health Care, but all failed. I became a practitioner in 2012 and did a few sessions on her. She is still here today. Her doctors were amazed, and to this day, they are not sure how it happened.

For so many, fear takes away the freedom of choice. But for me, life is about living, and living it to the fullest. I no longer use Band-Aids and I explore all of my Choices. If I had listened to my doctors when I was in my early 20s, I would not have my daughter, or my grandchildren.

January 2017, I lost the other most amazing woman in my life, my Mom. She was diagnosed with Lung Cancer and, once again, Fear played a factor in her decision as her doctors convinced her that removing the tumor was her only option. For two weeks she was cancer free, but then the worst thing imaginable hit, her cancer metastasized. You see, mom developed an infection right after the initial biopsy (which I tried to tell them) but was told I was not a doctor and they did not believe in intuition. How do you explain the symptoms that became apparent almost immediately after? The infection was already in her body before her surgery. We explored many choices afterward, but the infection overtook the cancer. The cancer treatments didn't work because of the infection, and the infection treatments didn't work because of the cancer.

That was another low point in my life, but instead of pills, drugs and alcohol, I instead used the tools in Alternative and Holistic Health Care that I had been exploring for the past 13 years. Reconnective Healing® is among the many Choices out there in Alternative and Holistic Health Care. For many of my clients, Reconnective

Healing® has been the start of their journey in exploring their Choices!

I know in my heart, had my grandmother and mother explored all their Choices and not let Fear make their decisions for them, they would still be here today.

October 9, 2017, I took another traumatic blow. I lost my house in the Tubbs Wildfire. My whole world was in there; all that was left of my family heirlooms, my mom and grandmother's possessions, just everything...my world as I knew it was my home, and all the things there were gone. Talk about staying numb, now I didn't even know who I was...I felt as if I lost my identity in the fire as well.

With losing my mom, and then the fire, I could have easily gone back to the day of wanting to stay numb by self-medicating with drugs and alcohol. But, thank God for all the Choices I have found these past 13 years. Western Medicine kept me sick and my Choices in Alternative and Holistic Health Care gave me my life back.

And so, the little girl who told stories, goes on to heal herself and others!

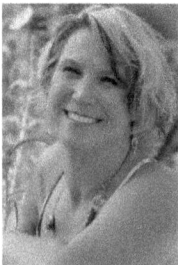

Cherri Gregori-Pedrioli was born and raised in beautiful Sebastopol, California and is proud to be a Sonoma County native. She started her career in the construction industry in the early 1980's. In 2004 she and her husband Duane founded Custom Plumbing and together they have created a very successful company.

Cherri's passion has always been helping others. Several years ago, while seeking alternatives to western medicine she was introduced to Reconnective Healing®. After her own amazing experiences, she decided in 2012 to start her own practice, Reconnect Mind Body Soul in Santa Rosa to offer Reconnective Healing to those who were also exploring energy healing as an alternative or addition to their current health care.

After the loss of both her beloved grandmother and mother, Cherri started on a mission to bring awareness and education in alternative and holistic health care to the community. She wants to get the message out that people have Choices that should be explored before making any life-changing decisions regarding their health.

Cherri was the first founding President of the Santa Rosa Holistic Chamber of Commerce. She is the founder of Holistic Choices Inc which includes Holistic Choices Network and along with Choices the Book Series and Co-Founder of Sonoma Strong Healing Fairs.

Cherri is the proud mother of John and Jeanie, stepmother to Nathan, Brandon and Sheanna and loving grandmother of six beautiful grandchildren. Her family is her greatest joy. Cherri enjoys spending time with her family, friends, boating, camping and the beach.

www.CherriPedrioli.com

Chapter 4

Arising from Victimhood to Forgiveness

by Angela Legh

"Unforgiveness is like a poison and a bitterness in your soul, and your life will always be bitter until you get rid of that poison." Joyce Meyers

When something bad happens to you, you have two choices...you can either decide to be a victim of the circumstances, or you can take responsibility for everything and everyone in your world. The choice you make can affect the outcome of the event, as well as color the rest of your life.

When I was twenty, I met, and quickly married, the man with whom I chose to spend over thirty years of my life. He was stable, put me on a pedestal, and it seemed as if it was him and me against the world.

We lived in a bubble, the two of us, and I slowly let go of friends and distanced myself from family...we only needed each other. Little did I know that there was a dark side to these behaviors.

From the start of the emotionally abusive behavior, I blamed him. I saw myself as the innocent one, the victim of his anger and control. I spent thirty years being the victim, feeling like I had no choice, feeling like I walked on eggshells, afraid of causing an outburst of anger. I felt that my words would be twisted into nefarious messages that I never meant to say...that I had never even thought. I felt as if the smallest problems could be escalated into full blown crisis. In this marriage there was no such thing as "agreeing to disagree."

There are stories I could tell, but I have no interest in causing him embarrassment. What I do have interest in, is to show that being the victim means that you give up your power to the other person and take no responsibility for the issue. If you aren't responsible, there is no mechanism you can put into place to fix the issue.

After reading the book "Becoming the Narcissist Worst Nightmare" by Shahida Arabi, I was awakened to the dynamics of my marriage. The worst events of my life were revealed in these pages, described as if the author was there in the room with us. As I read, I kept thinking, "That is what happened to me!"

Though this book can open your eyes and give you the strength and information needed to leave a marriage like mine, it also supports and encourages the victimization of the person on the receiving end of narcissistic abuse. Books like these are quick to instill self-esteem in the victim by saying, "It is not your fault." There is a place for this, for I know as well as anyone how emotional abuse can erode your self-esteem. But this leaves no room for self-examination. These types of books can be beneficial to find the wherewithal to leave a bad situation. However, you are best served when you discard the victim role once you are out on your own.

When you stay in your role as the victim, growth is not likely to happen. You will continue the same behavior and can end up in a different relationship that has the same dynamics. For your sake, for your happiness, it is crucial for you to step out of the victim role and assume responsibility for your choices.

For me, understanding my role began with looking at the situation through a wider lens. I could not do this while I lived within the everyday drama of the relationship. Once I removed myself, I could look at our behaviors with equanimity, to see that each of us filled a role in our relationship.

My role was that of a victim. When I am in the victim role, things are done to me by others. I have no control and others make all the choices. Once I realized that I was playing the victim role, I examined why I would do that. After much introspection, I understood that my higher self, my spirit, had wanted to learn a lesson that could only be provided through living a life exposed to this sort of behavior. I realized that my spirit had chosen this situation in my life, and had made an agreement with his spirit, for us both to learn the lessons available to us in this marriage.

Further, I learned that love is expressed both negatively and positively. I had thought that the negative behaviors I experienced were evidence that my ex-husband did not really love me. My interpretation of what was not love included being excessively yelled at, being shut out in anger, and other behaviors. One of my teachers asked me what love was. I struggled for an answer, and she told me to imagine that my higher self took me by the hand and showed me what love was. In my mind's eye I saw several vignettes – a mother snuggling with her baby, a young couple running and holding hands, an elderly couple helping each other, a father screaming at his son – wait!! I balked and said, "That isn't love!" My teacher calmly asked me if my last statement was true. I considered, and answered that the father loved his son, and was frightened that the son would get hurt. His fear resulted in the passion behind his words. This was eye opening for me; I immediately knew that my ex-husband did love me, but his fear and frustration colored what he said to me. My inability to understand this during our marriage is part of the reason why the marriage failed.

I take responsibility for not setting boundaries. I take responsibility for not setting an expectation of respectful behavior. I take responsibility for thinking I could "fix" the problem if I just loved him enough. I take responsibility for allowing the behavior to continue for so many years. I take responsibility for adopting narcissistic retaliation to try to hurt him in the way I felt I was being hurt.

I have since forgiven myself for making some mistakes, and for my choices in our marriage. I forgave him for his behavior in the past. Although I forgave him for his past behavior, I still held fear over being victimized again. This fear meant that I had more healing to do.

In the words of my good friend Janet Caliri, "Know that forgiveness is not about giving power TO someone, it is about TAKING BACK personal power/ownership...Forgiving is NOT about abdicating someone's behavior; it is about healing yourself...Additionally, forgiving yourself FIRST is the most crucial and compassionate step you can take." This philosophy, of taking back your power through forgiveness, is one that I have fully embraced.

I did some research on forgiveness, watched some Ted Talks, and accessed Lisa Nichol's Forgiveness series of videos. I eventually landed on the story of Dr. Hew Len, a psychiatrist assigned to work at an intensive psych ward in Hawaii in 1984. Dr. Len's story was told in a book entitled "Zero Limits", by Joe Dispenza and Dr. Len. When he started at the hospital, the scene was terrible, all of the patients were shackled, they were aggressive and unpredictable. The staff would walk with their backs to the wall, and they dreaded going to work. Dr. Len believed in ultimate responsibility, and so he believed that he was responsible for the patient's illness. He began performing a self-healing ritual called Ho'oponopono. He never met with patients, and he rarely left his office. He sat with the case files and practiced Ho'oponopono. Several months later, the aggression in the ward diminished. Patients were unshackled, and some were allowed outside. Staff began enjoying their jobs. Within three years, all patients were healed and released.

I began using the Ho'oponopono ritual, which includes the statements "I'm sorry, please forgive me, thank you, I love you", repeated over and over. This tool is the best way to forgive yourself, and through self-forgiveness, others in your sphere of influence can begin healing.

It was only through this ritual that I was fully committed to forgiving my ex-husband, as well as myself. I released the fear I had. I opened my heart and sent him loving energy. I communicated with him, clearly and effectively. I quit trying to fix him, and allowed him to be himself, without having to meet my expectations.

As I continue the practice of Ho'oponopono, I will continue to be healed. He can also be healed through my practice, because we are all connected. However, the goal is to self-heal, knowing that your healing is primary, for you are the creator of your reality. You are not trying to fix the other person, only yourself. This powerful practice can change your life, as well as the lives of those you love.

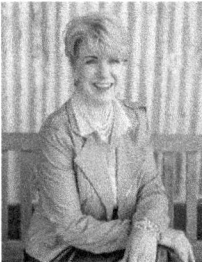

Angela Legh is sentient empath who, through adversity, felt the need to speak up. She became an author and speaker. Angela is intent on spreading light and love, making the world a better place. Through her company, Reveal Change, Angela strives to empower women to self-acceptance and self-love. Helping people to feel comfortable in their skin is a dream job for her!

Writing under a pen name, Angela wishes to keep the anonymity of individuals mentioned in her stories. She is writing her truth, and because of the duality of this world, her truth may not be the truth of the individuals featured in her story.

www.AngelaLegh.com

Chapter 5

The Magic of Jin Shin Jyutsu

by Deborah Myers

"Acupressure balances the body, mind, and spirit — empowering you to take charge of your own health." — Deborah Myers

That day seemed like any other day. I was driving through a residential neighborhood, looking forward to getting home after a long meeting with an insurance client. I put on my signal to change lanes and then — thwack! — my head hit the window. A moment later there was another thud as my head was thrown against the window again. That's the last thing I would remember about the accident for three months.

Although it took some time before I would understand the details of what happened, the accident was reverberating through my body, loud and clear. I was in constant pain, I suffered horrible headaches, and my neck and back were seriously inflamed. But I had to pay the bills, which meant working long hours in front of the computer, and on the phone, as well as hours in the car driving to clients' homes. Not only was my body under severe stress, my foggy mind made it close to impossible to keep up with the ever-growing must-do list.

What was especially hard, was the fact that I didn't feel on top of it with my kids and their schedules — homework, school events, special programs, sports. I was used to being 'team mom' for my son's soccer team, and I volunteered in the classroom several mornings a week. But so many things I had been used to doing, like rollerblading with the kids, were no longer options.

Despite the pain, I put on a stoic face and was able to take care of my work, home, and kids because, fortunately, for years I had been studying and practicing self-help acupressure. By doing a daily routine to balance my energy system, I was able to function, but I knew I needed an expert to help me fully heal. That's how I discovered Jin Shin Jyutsu, an ancient form of Japanese acupressure.

This gentle healing therapy strategically targeted critical acupressure points throughout my body, allowing it to release the inflammation and pattern of pain. I began to, once again, bend and move easily and enjoy all that my body could do. My clarity and focus improved. My productivity noticeably increased. My outlook became brighter.

That's when the light bulb came on. After years of chasing down the right career, I knew this was what I was meant to do. Jin Shin Jyutsu transformed me. It saved my body, my mind, and my spirit. I closed my insurance and securities office. I wanted to help others live more easily in their bodies too!

That was 1994, and I cannot imagine turning back the clock to do it differently. I am truly living my passion of helping others live healthier, happier, and more productive lives. For the last twenty-five years, I've been doing just that. Witnessing so many clients dramatically change how they are in their bodies has made my work so rewarding.

One of my early clients was Sara, a thirty-five-year-old mother of young children, who lived with excruciating neck pain and debilitating headaches. As a result, she often missed work and the quality of her life tanked. The doctors had diagnosed her with an inflammatory disease that was "irreversible" and the best she could hope for was to "contain the pain with medication."

Her situation was all too familiar, so I felt confident acupressure would help. Sara and I began working together to repattern her body to let go of inflammation and pain. As time progressed, Jin Shin Jyutsu allowed her easier, more flexible movement. Her emotions stabilized, and she was less reactive—able to handle stressful situations and anxiety in a much calmer way.

Now in her fifties, Sara enjoys a very full, active life. Thanks to the magic of Jin Shin Jyutsu, she was able to resume her nursing career. Today, her children, now in their twenties and thirties, look back on a happy childhood playing softball, backpacking, and biking with their mother.

While I was giving Sara one-on-one Jin Shin Jyutsu treatments, I also spent time teaching her self-help acupressure. Daily practice helped her always stay ahead of the pain. She applied what she learned to help her children. With her encouragement, as well as that from many other clients, I was inspired to create a series of workshops to teach self-help acupressure.

I wanted to show people how to be partners with their own bodies. Non-intrusive and gentle, Jin Shin Jyutsu replenishes mental, physical, and emotional energy, and allows breathing to be more expansive. Where energy flows, the breath follows. It seems like magic: it can reduce stress, balance emotions, improve performance, increase clarity and focus, and strengthen self-confidence and mindfulness. When we target pressure points to relieve bothersome symptoms and maintain energy balance, it's very empowering.

For the last twenty-five years, I have taught all my clients a nine-step self-help acupressure routine called 'The Daily Clean Your House Flow®'. As time went by, I wanted children to have an easy way to learn and experience energy balancing that was fun, so I created an animated video of the Daily Flow.

After Joey, a third grader, told me why he was doing the Daily Flow several times a day, I was convinced how important it is to empower children with a way they can affect how they feel. He told me studying was easier, so he was getting better grades. He told me that he was even getting along better with his brother and, he said, "That's crazy!" The Daily Flow was making a difference in people's lives.

Kristen was a highly motivated sixteen-year-old. She carried an intense load of classes, as well as pursued sports, music, and community service — all of which she felt were necessary to receive the scholarships she was hoping for. But anxiety creeped in, affecting her sleep, her grades, her sense of well-being, and her emotional stability. Understandably, her parents were worried and sought out help. Receiving Jin Shin Jyutsu treatment, and practicing self-help acupressure, allowed Kristen to break through the anxiety, the fear, and the worry. She graduated with honors, loves being at college, and now Kristen has tools she can rely on. "Whenever I have feelings come up that I don't understand, I just do my energy work and I feel better," she says.

Stress affects the energetic balance of the body systems, as does trauma. In fall 2017, thousands of people in Sonoma County experienced trauma, beyond description, as they raced away from the blazing infernos that had been their homes. The impact from those few days of hell, left emotional scars, particularly for youngsters.

I used Jin Shin Jyutsu to help Justin, a five-year-old who could not understand why he had lost his belongings, why he didn't have his old bedroom to go home to, and why his cat was no longer part of the family. He was suffering a physical shortness of breath from smoke inhalation, plus his breath had been taken away by the trauma. This caused him to be more and more stuck in the memory and sadness, and he was plagued by recurring nightmares. As I applied gentle touch on energy meridian points, his lungs opened to release the buildup of smoke, his body remembered the old pattern of expansive breath, he broke through the nightmares, and he started smiling and laughing again.

Why did the energy balancing of Jin Shin Jyutsu help Justin and his parents begin their healing and get their breath back after the fires? It's energy that makes us tick! Every single one of us is made up of energy, and energy is meant to flow. It's energy that helps all our systems — respiratory, digestive, vascular, muscular, skeletal — work individually and concurrently so our bodies can function easily and effortlessly.

We can access that energy by placing fingertips on designated points to harmonize and restore the energy flow. Holding these points in combination, releases accumulated tension, and resets the body to its natural state of balance. Our bodies are miracles. When mind, body, and spirit are in balance, we are able to tap into the wisdom of the body, interpret the messages, and restore harmony. The body is brought back to its full potential.

Jin Shin Jyutsu helped Sara, Justin, Joey, and Kristen release tension and pain by balancing and replenishing mental, physical, and emotional energies. Acupressure transformed their lives, and it transformed mine. I feel blessed to be able to bring the magic of Jin Shin Jyutsu to those who need to release stuck energy. And the best part, is that this ancient acupressure is something we can each do for ourselves. It empowers us with the understanding that health is at our fingertips, and it gives us the ability to take charge of our own well-being.

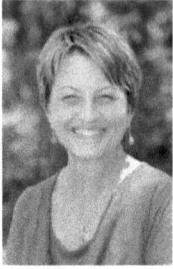

A certified Acupressurist and Jin Shin Jyutsu practitioner, Deborah helps people get and stay healthy. Since 1995, she has worked one-on-one with clients utilizing light, gentle touch to reduce stress, relieve pain, and bring balance to body, mind, and spirit.

Deborah is on a mission to teach others how they can be partners with their own bodies. She founded Deborah Myers Wellness to treat, educate, inspire, and empower people of all ages to achieve balance and integrated health.

To share the magic of acupressure, Deborah developed the Easy Self-Help Acupressure Program for kids in classrooms and in their homes. The program includes an animated video of the Daily Clean Your House Flow®, a nine-step self-help acupressure flow, and an accompanying book. Kids, parents, and teachers are finding that following the program increases clarity and focus, reduces anxiety, balances emotions, increases mindfulness, and enhances daily activities. Posters and instructional videos are also available.

Through one-on-one Jin Shin Jyutsu treatments, coaching, workshops, workplace wellness programs, and her Easy Self-Help Acupressure video and books, Deborah has helped thousands of people of all ages discover how they can take charge of their own health. Learn more about her work at

www.DeborahMyersWellness.com

Chapter 6

Downward Spiral

by Janet Caliri

*"Want What You Have and Don't Want What You
Do Not Have!"*

At the bus stop, I feel excitement, coupled with expectation and longing. Interestingly enough, I also feel anxious, almost a foreboding. I need the help of a familiar friend, like my cousin. But somehow it almost seems too simple…when I approach Boston and family, nothing ever remains simple.

And that's when my cell phone rings. I'm almost terrified to look at the display. My stomach begins to churn.

So, I peek.

Oh shit. It's Mom. This can't be good; somehow, she's going to jump in and make this challenging time worse. Nonetheless, I answer. She says with that familiar martyr tone "I spoke with your Aunt who told me she questioned you and your cousins' arrangement. Well, you're not staying with her, you're coming home to stay with your Father and me."

"This is none of your friggin' business - it's between me and my cousin." I hear myself say, with anger and resentment.

The whole 5-hour overnight flight to Boston involves swollen eyes and another sleepless night at 35,000 feet. No appetite. Could not hold a thought. Just furious. Furious when I needed to be curious. I am a fucking adult. An adult in trouble. An adult with something undiagnosed…an unknown illness. But an adult, nonetheless. What gives them the right to interfere with me and my cousin?! Oh, that's right, the need to control! I claim my power by telling my truth. Every day. From this moment forward...

I don't remember the landing, or how I got to my parents' house. But I am here, sitting across from them tired, and screaming in my parents' living room. The last couch I slept on was despair, this one is screaming. Standing up to them, saying things they do not want to hear. It is not well received. Telling them they don't know WHAT I need! And they aren't even trying to find out — they are just imposing whatever oversimplified theory they think will give them the most direct route to resolving their own embarrassment about their adult daughter's struggle and dependency. I feel insulted. Somehow disagreeing or disappointment with my choices, notions and reasons, means that they're right and I'm wrong? A worthwhile relationship is impossible without truth and transparency.

I am distraught. Despite that I refuse to surrender my personal power, even in the face of my weakness, and my admission of it. I am NOT subscribing to their false story — not to avoid conflict. Not to expedite fulfillment of my basic needs. I'm just not.

Why bother living?

Wailing and flailing on the floor of my childhood bedroom, eyes locked on the round rug, I recall life is not linear. Now staring at the hardwood floors, and stark white walls thru puffy eyes, I seek solace in my warm fuzzy clothes on my back.

Its daylight. Through blurry eyes, I notice the pink swirls on the white rug, spiraling around me. I feel like I've been wrenching for hours, bawling my eyes out. My tongue feels like a toxic stew of trash coming out of my mouth...I recall, life is not linear.

How did I get here? I don't want to think about it anymore. It's been days, or weeks, or longer...I'm so done with it! Done with everything. Where is my motivation to get off this floor - to go to the next floor… to do anything? I've known my purpose, and I always thought that would be enough. But it is not. How can that not be enough? If it's true that it's not enough, what does that mean? What's next? Here I am, sick…years into adulthood, and on the floor of my childhood bedroom…and I don't know where I'm going to get the motivation to heal. And live.

Like a tube of toothpaste having its insides squeezed out, I surrender to this moment. I am humbled. Dear Life, "What?! What will motivate me to move forward, to heal and be of service once again? Because at this juncture, I am done with life, yet I know the muted spark remains, so…what the fuck?!" I drop the question into a pink bubble on its way into the ethers. I go on with my days.

Days go by, and yet again I'm on the floor. I don't want to be here, but this seems to be where the answers come. This is a safe place in some regards, and I have a roof over my head. In a state of curiosity and connection with the Universe, the answer whispers in my ear…CREATION. "What!? Creation? Ok, thanks and SO WHAT?!, Now what?!" This abiding in the state of curiosity is working well, so I leave the question again.

What feels like an exorbitant amount of time, the ethers finally nudged me with a pop-up command: *Take pictures of your emotions. All of them, not just the ones you like.* Happily, I obeyed this command and asked myself, "Janet, what does anger look like? What does relief look like? What does compassion look like?" Clicking away, making abstract, symbolic, pantomimed and literal images, I am feeling free and expansive! Ah-ha moment…I am CREATING with curiosity and a camera!

I suddenly recognized that I am BEing WITH my emotions, in each moment, with each click! These energy forms that are meant to be simply observed, yet typically are met with resistance, now have NO power over me. I feel elated. I am entering sovereignty. I am reminding myself that E-motions are energy in motion and MUST move through us like a river or the wind. When I attempt to control them, by either pushing away, changing or attaching, I am creating blocks and scars in my energy body. Recalling that, over time, these often have led to my conditioned fears, limiting beliefs, and a variety of illnesses.

I recognized the imperative of this process. It is my ticket to freedom from illness and limiting beliefs, holding me back from my potential. I thought, "Life, you are too funny!" just a few months after publishing my first book, *Me With Me*, I was being tested on self-love, self-care, self-honor. Ha! I am my first client!

Reflection: From this story, I remind us all that we are always at choice. There are many options and possibilities at our fingertips. And curiosity leads the way.

During this trying time in my life, I was still curious, but I was in denial (of what I needed to do, just to live – feed myself, pay the bills, be healthy). So, there's a more sincere form of curiosity which I was not engaging, or I would have bypassed the denial.

I had determination, but it wasn't enough.

I had grit, but it wasn't enough. Those closest to me doubted my path at the time; despite this, I persevered.

I took ownership, but it wasn't enough.

I had innovation, but it wasn't enough.

So, the moral of the story, is that favorable outcomes follow to the degree I am abiding in sincere curiosity, and to the corresponding degree to which fear is disempowered. Telling ourselves the truth is easy, by playfully abiding in sincere curiosity.

Over the next two years, I received two more significant messages from the Universe. The second was, using a camera, track subtle evidences of my progress. The third was, using a camera, capture what triggers my emotions to significantly reduce the emotional charge.

I happily obeyed the instructions, which lead me to more ease, joy and personal power. Ultimately, this 3-part process was my saving grace! Allow me to introduce you to that grace, Visible Transitions!

Client example: A mother and her 9-year-old daughter lost their home and private school to the October 2017 wildfires here in Sonoma County. I took them on a photo-walk-about and asked the girl what she values in friendship. One value was 'acceptance' so I asked her "What does acceptance look like?" Typically, most people respond with "I don't know" as did she, so we continued to walk. Suddenly she came up with an idea and photographed that. After a few moments, she began to mildly shake, with her teeth chattering uncontrollably. Her mom and I met eyes knowing she was having a somatic release of trauma!

Client example: a lovely woman working for the county and I began working together in my Visible Transitions program just a few months after her home burnt to the ground, in the October 2017 Sonoma Wildfires. During our very first session, without having said anything directly, I instinctively knew she was in an unhealthy [verbally abusive] marriage. As we journeyed through my program, her stress and overwhelm subsided, her confidence and personal boundaries developed, thus began to make difficult choices that were ultimately for the benefit of all beings. She was loving herself in a way she had not previously, by finding her voice. Some of her people were uncomfortable with that. Regardless, she moved forward in a way that aligned with her true nature. She's now a published author, is closing in on being officially divorced, funding projects dear to her heart, left her job that was not aligned with her values, and traveling the world, immersing in further personal transformation with like-hearted folk. Now that is what I call evidence of progress and a visible transition!

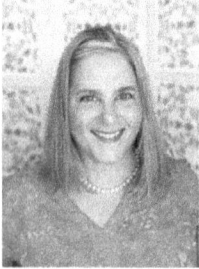

Janet Caliri is a creative, energetic and sought-after international speaker, author and coach who brings her innovative and playful process to audiences across the nation. Participants at her events laugh, wonder and explore their childlike curiosity as they discover the keys for ease in life transitions. She has helped thousands of people examine the role of images for effective change and walk away with the tools to go from Stress to Ease, Fear to Personal Power, and Anxiety to Productivity in their own life transitions.

Her vast experience as a former cardiovascular radiology tech, professional photographer, certified life coach, published author, and trained youth artist teacher are the secret to her client's transformation. Their transformation is two- fold: They develop emotional intelligence and navigate their days from playful curiosity rather than emotional reactivity, by simply using a smart phone camera!

Survivors of trauma, youth, under-served populations, and professional Mom's feel empowered by creating imagery of their emotions, acknowledging the subtleties of their progress, and dissolving their conditioned stories. Thus, they become more present, connected and productive while de-escalating stress and trauma.

Janet is not only the founder of Visible Transitions; she is a product of her product having overcome her own overwhelming transmutations. Real change happens as Janet introduces childlike wonder into her private sessions, and dynamic events, as participants discover the secrets to building bridges from where they are to where we want to be.

www.JanetCaliri.com

Chapter 7

Motivation to Change

by Karen & Rob Wagner

"A journey of a thousand miles begins with a single step."– Lao Tzu

Karen's story: After my parents' ugly divorce, my father secretly relocated my younger sister and me from a small town in Illinois to Southern California on what we thought was a vacation to Disneyland. Being taken away from our friends and family, my sister and I became best friends, and we looked out for and supported each other through some very difficult times as we were growing up.

I remember feeling confused, angry and abandoned most of the time. Self-doubt and mistrust guided most of my young thought processes. To cope, I adopted many unhealthy habits over the years as a means to regulate my emotions.

Unhealthy thinking led to making some pretty poor life-choices. Body image issues led to eating disorders, including unhealthy dieting and binge eating. A need for belonging led to unhealthy partying, and my desire to feel loved led to unhealthy relationships. In short, I surrendered control over my own life looking for love, security, and happiness outside of myself. Then one day, I realized there had to be something more, so decided to get my own apartment in California and make a new life.

One night, an invitation from my best friend would change everything in my world.

Rob's story: I grew up in a very small town in Michigan with three sisters. Life was comfortable and predictable. We lived in the same house, went to same school and had the same friends, from kindergarten through high school.

During my childhood, my mom was very ill, always in and out of hospitals, and my dad worked multiple jobs to take care of the family, so we didn't see them much. My sisters and I would take care of most of the household chores and watched out for each other. We learned to be self-sufficient at a very early age.

By the age of 18, I was working in a factory, like most everyone else in my hometown. My life consisted of working all week and partying all weekend. I thought this was the way life was supposed to be. Then one day, I realized there had to be something more, so I decided to move to California to make a new life.

One night, an invitation from my best friend would change everything in my world.

Our story: So, how do soulmates find each other? At a dance club called 'Mississippi Moonshine', of course! On that night, a young Michigan boy walked up and introduced himself to a young California girl with the most beautiful eyes he had ever seen—and, in the wink of an eye, both lives would be changed forever. To this day, we still dispute who was checking who out first. Unbeknownst to us at the time, God had a plan for us that started long before we met in that dance club that night. This would be the night everything in our lives would change forever.

We married a year and a half later, and the early years of marriage were not perfect, by any means. We started a business, and quickly learned our lack of vision, experience and discipline, would prove to be a lethal combination. Disappointed, but not defeated, we changed course and moved to a new town and started new jobs. A change we affectionately dubbed "Operation Simple."

As our new life started to unfold, we would soon be blessed with our first child. All seemed to be going great until one day, after experiencing severe pain during the second trimester, test results revealed that I had a very large mass on my ovaries. The doctors were concerned that it could be cancer, and decided I needed surgery as soon as possible. However, nothing could be done until the baby was mature enough to survive the surgery. Fear and anxiety dominated our lives for the next 3 months, until the baby was strong enough to survive on his own after the surgery, if necessary. By the grace of God, the tumor was benign, and miraculously our son arrived into the world, safe and sound. Just 18 months later, our beautiful daughter arrived, with her own special flare, on New Year's Eve.

I stayed home with the kids before they started school while Rob worked three jobs to support us. We thought we were doing what was best for our family. Actually, it would be the start of what would become a very unhealthy work-life balance for Rob, and it affected our family in many ways for years to come. Company closings, and forced relocations, seemingly plagued our early years. Eventually, we would be led back to Northern California to continue our journey with our family.

When the kids were old enough to start school, I decided to take a job working for the school district so I could be home with the kids on their schedule. At the time, it was a job of convenience, but it turned out to be a rewarding career spanning over two decades as a Special Educational Assistant to children of all ages with moderate to severe disabilities. It's been such a blessing to have a small part in helping these special kids learn how to live better and more productive lives.

All our hard work began to pay off and our careers were advancing. Unfortunately, a series of life-changing events would come to dominate our lives. My 61-year old birth mother fell unexpectedly ill and was hospitalized. As a complete shock, she was diagnosed with inoperable cancer and given only a few days to live. While at her bedside, my younger sister had a grand-mal seizure in the ICU room and was admitted to the same hospital that night. The next day, a CTE scan revealed my sister had inoperable brain cancer. My mother would lose her battle a few days later and we took my sister home with us to seek treatment and care for her. My beautiful sister would lose her battle, too, just 8 weeks later at the age of 38. No words will ever convey the shock, sorrow, and loss we feel to this day.

Soon after the loss of my sister, my father and my stepmother's health began to rapidly deteriorate, due primarily to very unhealthy habits and very poor diets. My father was morbidly obese, and my stepmother required dialysis caused from diabetes-related kidney failure. We became their primary caregivers for the next several years, while managing our own young family.

While focusing most of our attention on the care of others for so many years, we stopped taking care of ourselves, and we became stressed-out workaholics with very unhealthy habits of our own. We both would become obese, with a host of health-related issues.

One day, by the grace of God, we reconnected with an old friend we hadn't seen in many years, and we noticed he and his wife both had amazing health transformations. That was the day a health program was shared with us that changed everything.

Our friends became our personal health coaches and taught us how to change our habits. We started our health journey together, with their guidance. With our newfound healthy habits, our weight steadily dropped, and our health dramatically improved.

Things were going great on our health journey, until one day; I became aware something was off with the way I felt and went to the doctor. I would soon discover I had a rare cancer, needed to have emergency surgery, and undergo chemotherapy treatments for the next 5-months.

My doctors needed my weight to remain steady, so my body could tolerate the chemotherapy treatments. With my coaches help, we modified my food plan to keep my weight as steady as possible throughout my treatment. I successfully completed the treatments with very little weight change, and very few side-effects. My success was due to a result of my healthier lifestyle and the help a dear friend provided, as my personal reconnective energy-healing practitioner. Today, I'm cancer-free and living life with a completely new perspective. We give God all the glory for saving my life, and we give our health program, and our commitment to live better lives, the credit for transforming our physical, mental and financial health.

Through all our trials, we realized our true passion was helping others. So, we became certified health coaches and dedicated our lives to the pursuit of helping other people live their best lives, too. The blessings on this journey have been too many to count.

We take great joy in teaching people how to shift their mindset and develop better habits. Today, we work together as a coaching team, helping other people find joy and learn to live their best lives. We are living proof that it's never too late to find your purpose, passion, and joy, as long as you are still alive.

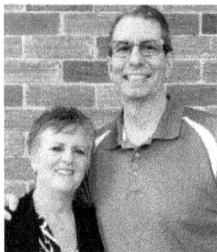

Rob & Karen Wagner have been married since 1986 and reside in the beautiful wine country of Sonoma County, California. They have two grown children living in Northern California as well.

Rob has been a food manufacturing executive since 1998. Karen has been a paraprofessional special ed assistant, working with handicapped children since 1998. They are active with their local church and community.

Rob and Karen, each lost over 80 lbs. and Rob stopped taking three weight-related medications while both dramatically improved their health, and in doing so, realized they needed to share what they learned and became certified health coaches through the MacDonald Center for Obesity Prevention and Education. They have since dedicated their lives to their own health and the health and well-being of others.

www.RobandKarenWagner.com

Chapter 8
I Found Freedom
by Maghen Ward

*"When I don't know who I am, I serve you. When I
know who I am, I am you."*

There are alternatives to medicine and doctors. Medicine is what we take while the body heals itself. My parents worked day and night to give our family a comfortable life. They lived a life dedicated to helping others, usually at their own expense. Meanwhile, I was bullied at school by a group of girls who singled me out for being the preppy, good girl with money. The 12-year combat with these girls, some sexual abuse and losing friends to murder and accidents really motivated me to become a private investigator in order to fight the bad guys.

I opened up my private detective firm when I was 23. I had to learn how to handle all the persecution that came with being a young female investigator with no law enforcement background, entering into a male dominated sector. Experiencing this, and the work itself, created a cynic out of me, but the hardships did not stop there. I had many unhealthy romantic relationships over my lifetime which took up most of my time and energy. Due to this distraction, the death of my best friend came as a surprise to me. He was sick and I did not know until it was too late.

After the death of my best friend in 2015, I felt empty, and I had suffered enough. I decided to stop working immediately and begin a search for the meaning of life. But I didn't know where to start, and my mathematical brain would not allow for any spiritual endeavors. I was on the verge of giving up on life. So, I decided to accept an open invitation to a wedding in Hawaii and just go where the wind would take me.

While on my trip, I decided to stay focused on me and work to remain happy in every moment. In turn, I felt I elevated my level of consciousness. This was the beginning of my transformation.

Looking back now, I am able to recall that I was entering into a 'Jhana', or a state of prolonged meditation, concentration, and stillness, where my mind was fully immersed in staying happy. Or, in other words, I found God. Or, most likely, I finally allowed myself to feel the love of God.

The bliss I felt grew. Up until I couldn't really feel the heavy state of my body anymore; everything felt light. I didn't know what was going on, nor did I care. I wanted to take this bliss that I felt one step further. Since I couldn't feel the heaviness of my body anymore, I wondered how it would react under heightened circumstances. I took a hot shower and I couldn't feel the heat; I stuck my hand in the fire of the barbecue, and no harm was done. I began to have the ability to alter my body temperature, and my confidence was increasing. By the end of the trip, I had levitated off of the ground. This was the peak of the experience. I experienced this spiritual awakening in every cell of my being, to the point where all I knew was light. Upon returning to California, I gave away everything I owned, and I went out to seek knowledge around the USA. This had turned into a full-fledged spiritual investigation of who I was and what the world around me is. Slowly I began to follow the teachings of Christ and started to realize that it was His Love for me that is responsible for these happenings.

I began practicing fasting and prayer. I did a 3-day, 5-day, 8-day and 40-day fast. During these fasts, I began to tap into other gifts that I had been given. One night, I dreamt of healing others with a touch of my hand. The next morning when I went out to the store, I saw a woman who couldn't lift her feet off of the ground. I asked her if I can touch her and say a few words. After doing this three times, she was able to walk normally. She thanked me and looked very grateful. I soon found myself looking forward to seeing injured people in order to help them.

Miracles are just events that science cannot explain yet. They continue on in my life. My experiences made me realize that in order to save the world, I had to use love instead of power. I realized that the bad guy had never been the person, but rather the fear that drove each person. Therefore, in order to fight evil, I had to give love. So, I had to recreate my life's plan to help humanity. Love is what healed that woman. My new goal became to teach people that anything is possible, and a life without suffering is right around the corner. We are all born perfect and happy, and it's what we choose to do, that brings us suffering. If we cut those things out, we create a happier life.

I am a daughter of God. His love saved me from myself. I love God/Love with all my Heart, Mind and Soul. When you love something, you become one with it. All the wrongs in this world are there to teach us how to make the world right. It has taken me 28 years to realize that Unconditional Love is who I am. Peace, love, compassion, kindness, surrendering, patience. I spend most of my time in prayer. I am. We are One. I heard a calling to discover myself in 2016. Now, I have fully realized. Now, I am blessed to walk it out. Loving Awareness. As Ram Dass says, "Let's all walk each other home."

Along my journey, I learned one very important thing; there is nothing that suffering can offer us. The only way to energize ourselves is through love. We should love, not because it is the right thing to do, but because it creates enough energy inside you to make anything possible.

Jesus is the way and the truth and the light.

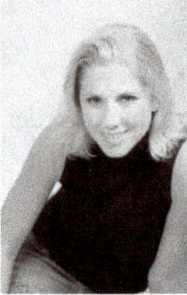

Maghen Ward is a Private investigator, Hypnotherapist, Life Coach, Author and Speaker with a Mathematical background from Sonoma State University. She owns and operates Wards Investigations and Legal Services in California. During her rigorous times as a detective, she underwent a spiritual transformation and awakening. Some people refer to it as being saved. She is now ready to spread the good news that this transformation has brought to her.

Maghen has dedicated her life to unconditional love and is helping others broaden their level of awareness. Her focus remains on practices that help awaken our minds, bodies and spirits.

www.MaghenWard.com

Chapter 9
Can the Impossible Be Possible?
by Patrice Fistor-Jaehnig

*"We are slowed down sound and light waves, a
walking bundle of frequencies tuned into the
cosmos. We are souls dressed up in sacred
biochemical garments and our bodies are the
instruments through which our souls play their
music." - Albert Einstein*

At age 15, I'm in front of my orthopedic surgeon who tells me he
wants to put me into a contraption called a "Milwaukee Brace"
immediately. I refuse because I don't want to be considered a "freak"
at school.

I had been diagnosed with severe scoliosis. I had a 29-degree "S"
curve, with a rotation so that my right shoulder was dropped and
curved forward to accommodate for the curve in my back. My right
back rib cage protruded out so much more than the left that I could
not even sit in a chair with both sides of my back touching it. My left
hip was significantly torqued to the left.

I chose to work very hard with a Physical Therapist, religiously
doing my exercises twice a day. I wore a lift in my right shoe, had
something under my left hip when sitting, would lie down as much
as possible to counter the effect of gravity, and made many other
adjustments in my life to keep the curve from increasing. I was right-
handed and had to learn to do things such as bowling, throwing a
softball, and doing a tennis serve with my left hand. I had x-rays
taken every four to six weeks and the doctor told me that, if my
curve increased one degree, I was going into that brace. That was
incentive enough for me, and I actually decreased that curve by a

degree, to the amazement of my orthopedist. However, the scoliosis continued to be problematic for me.

Years later, because of my disability, I was trained as a Certified Shorthand Reporter, supported by the State of California. That career was stressful emotionally, as well as challenging physically. It entailed sitting for long periods and, as time went on, the scoliosis became more and more uncomfortable. The emotional stress arose from the sometimes violent, ugly family law or criminal cases, the high-strung attorneys, and the consistently negative legal environment. The physical challenge was obvious and increasing from the continuous typing and sitting. Eventually, I was prescribed pain and sleep medications just to function. Chronic pain, when treated with drugs, creates feelings of depression and hopelessness. It was unbearable to go on living in such pain and stress. I was determined to find another way to heal myself.

In February 2000, I found myself at a healing seminar in San Francisco. The Instructor, Dr. Eric Pearl, had asked the audience for volunteers who had a visible deformity to join him on the stage so that he could demonstrate the specific energy/frequency healing that he was teaching, now known as Reconnective Healing. Another woman and I both had scoliosis, and amazingly, had very similar limitations in range of motion. Neither of us could reach our right hand around to our back.

We were standing at the front of the seminar room. Dr. Pearl was standing between us, moving his hands around us, not touching us, except for sometimes lightly touching our shoulders. He was speaking with the audience as he did this, not really focusing on me or the other woman. I had been very skeptical about the possibility of waving ones' hands in the air to effect miraculous healing results, so when, about 10 minutes later he asked the other woman to demonstrate whether she had any increase in her range of motion and she showed no demonstrable increase, I thought, "I knew it! This is a bunch of baloney. I can wave my hands in the air and, Poof! someone gets a healing? Yeah, right."

Then it was my turn to show if I had a significant change.

"Oh, my God!" I gasped, as I was able to raise my right arm up behind my back, an increase of more than six inches in a movement that I never remembered being able to do. It felt like my body had realigned itself. Even more remarkably, the chronic pain I had been experiencing for 30 years was gone!

It was through a series of synchronicities, which I now believe were orchestrated by the Universe, that I ended up at this seminar. And, little did I know, that weekend would totally change the trajectory of my life.

In addition to learning how to facilitate Reconnective Healing for myself and others, I also went on to learn and teach another application of the Reconnective Healing frequencies of energy, light and information called "The Personal Reconnection."

Before learning to offer this to others, I was required to experience it myself. I was told I would be reconnecting a gridwork of lines and points on my body to an infinite structure, connecting me more fully to the energetics of the earth, star systems and interdimensionally. It was supposed to put me back on my own life course, ready or not. I'd heard that others had amazing experiences during this process, and I expected something dramatic to happen to me on the massage table when I had this two-session, once-in-a-lifetime, process facilitated. For both sessions, on consecutive days, I lay there with my eyes closed, in anticipation, and did not feel a thing. For all I knew, the practitioner could have left and gone for coffee and returned 40 minutes later to tap me on the shoulder and "bring me back." From where?

If the prior physical healing had not occurred at that seminar, I would have thought there was nothing to this; that it wasn't real. However, about four months later I had an "ah-ha" moment when I realized that, since having the Personal Reconnection, my way of being and my life had changed dramatically.

I recognized that in the previous months numerous issues or problems that I had been avoiding for years had come right in front of me again, and instead of resisting, I had moved through them. I realized that I had been living and acting out of fear, and now the fear was falling away. It seemed that anything was possible moving forward. Maybe something had happened after all!

I began assisting at Dr. Pearl's seminars and eventually left my court reporting career to develop a healing practice locally and to travel with Dr. Pearl and The Reconnection's worldwide Teaching Team. I travelled to over 60 cities in about 30 countries around the globe during the next 15 years.

I've been honored to witness hundreds of seemingly miraculous healings during those travels, as well as in my own practice. Some of these have been physical, such as actually seeing bones lengthen; tumors move, shrink or even disappear; "terminal" diseases have ceased to exist, infertile women were able to conceive, chronic pain was relieved, clients' feelings of well-being and wholeness returned.

Though I never can predict if, when, or how results from a session may manifest, and cannot make any promises or guarantees, I truly know a healing on some level occurs for every client. Sometimes it's obvious to them immediately; sometimes it unfolds over time. Occasionally, the client doesn't even realize that the shifts that have taken place within them are related to their Reconnective Healing or Personal Reconnection sessions.

I recently had a client come in complaining of hip problems and difficulty walking. After our session, she felt some relief, but was still in some discomfort. A few weeks later I received a call from her. She hadn't told me previously that a sonogram, taken prior to her seeing me, had shown a 60% occlusion of the main artery in her left kidney. She had just recently received results from her latest sonogram showing no appreciable occlusion. Her kidney was functioning at 100% capacity. She was calling to tell me that she now knows the healing was not solely for what she was anticipating, her hip; but more vitally, her kidney function.

Currently, I am back in Northern California enjoying my profession as a Reconnective Healing Foundational and Reconnection Certified Practitioner, Practitioner Mentor and an Associate Instructor of The Reconnection. I'm grateful that Reconnective Healing found me, leading me to discover my true-life path and passion and to change my career completely. My practice is called *Heartlight Healing*. I offer consultations, Reconnective Healing sessions in person or by distance, and the evolutionary process called 'The Personal Reconnection'.

While science continues to explore how it works, Reconnective Healing has been documented in more than a dozen international studies. Reconnective Healing allows the client to return to an optimal state of balance on multiple levels, including physical, mental, emotional and/or spiritual. When we entrain with the Reconnective Healing Frequencies of energy, light, and information we emit more biophotons and vibrate at a higher level of light. Studies have shown that this can also restructure our DNA. When these frequencies are introduced, they create coherence and order, greater harmony, and reconnect our entire being to our greatest human potential.

Had my scoliosis not changed so dramatically that day in 2000, I would not have believed what I thought was impossible was even possible. Now I know that we are limitless, and the possibilities for healing and transformation are endless.

Reconnective Healing has changed thousands of lives and I plan to make sure it changes many more!

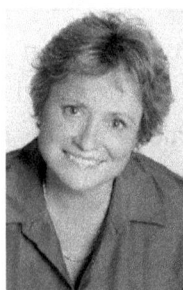

Patrice Fistor-Jaehnig is an Internationally recognized Foundational Practitioner of Reconnective Healing®, The Reconnection-Certified Practitioner®, Practitioner Mentoring, and Associate Instructor of The Reconnection®.

I worked for over 23 years in the highly demanding legal system as a court reporter and experienced numerous health challenges. Traditional medical care and drugs were not the solution for me, so I looked for alternative choices, which led to my discovery of Reconnective Healing and The Reconnection.

Since late 2000, I've traveled throughout the world teaching and assisting at seminars to bring Reconnective Healing and The Reconnection to as many people on the planet as possible. I am honored to have shared this with thousands worldwide and to also serve my own community. I am facilitating my clients' interaction with a comprehensive bandwidth of frequencies of energy, light and information which bring about the appropriate changes for the client at that time to more fully connect with their full potential and perfection. Changes may occur on multiple levels – physical, mental, emotional and spiritual. I currently have private practices in two locations located about an hour north of San Francisco in Santa

Rosa, and Windsor, California. I also offer distance healing and love doing healing for animals, as well.

Please contact me for a free consultation to learn more about Reconnective Healing and the two-session, once-in-a-lifetime process of The Personal Reconnection. Your future awaits, and I await hearing from you!

www.PatriceFistorJaehnig.com

Chapter 10

The Power of Light and Sound Therapy and the Use of Crystals

by Simon Emsley, PhD

"You realize you are part of the hologram of life, surrounded by an aura or energy field that radiates distinct colour and vibrations. The aura fingertips your soul and reflects your goodness, wellness, mental stability, maturity, emotional/inner turmoil or peaceful fulfilment. More of each of these qualities, peace, wellness, stability, maturity and fulfilment may become your ever-present precious possession by the application of color's power in our daily living." ~ Morton Walker

There are many life changing events that occur along our life paths. Some are small, others are of monumental proportions. At each step, as each event unfolds, we are given choices…some are mundane; "What sort of coffee should I buy?" Others are of critical importance; "Should I accept the chemotherapy treatment or not? What are the odds of lengthening my life compared with the side effects and quality of life?" Other choices may be; "Should I have a knee replacement or stem cell regeneration therapy to reduce the pain in my knees?" For a friend of mine, he had no choice; he had pulmonary arterial hypertension; he had to use an oxygen supply until he could get a lung transplant. You will see that in these few lines, the choices focus on Conventional Western Medicine. This book, and these chapters, focus on the alternative therapies that are available as complementary or integrative methods.

For me, the life changing event was less dramatic, perhaps. After thirty years working in Industry, I was laid off in, at that time, the latest Oil Price Crash. The crash was caused by the vagaries of the capital markets, politics, capitalism, and the cyclical nature of the Oil and Gas business. The price of a barrel of oil crashed from a peak of $115 per barrel in June 2014 to under $35 by the end of February 2016. It was one of the most important global macroeconomic developments, and many hundreds of thousands of people lost their jobs, and rig count plummeted. Both myself and my partner survived in our oil exploration positions through three rounds of layoffs but were caught by the fourth. We were given choices; to stay in Houston and find new positions or follow a long-held desire to establish a place to help others. The founders were presented with the opportunity to start down the path of developing the Iaso Wellness Center.

Our mission is to facilitate life changing transformations for our clients through our uniquely integrated approach to energy and vibrational therapeutic methods. We use vibrational energy therapies to help reduce stress, anxiety, and chronic issues, such as pain. These issues can be debilitating, causing insomnia, issues at work including lack of productivity. These also affect your relationships and love; for yourself and others. We help reduce these issues by balancing your energy and life force so that you can live a more productive and fulfilling life. Our methods work on past and present issues and traumas so that you can create a fabulous future.

I am an Energy Practitioner and mainly use Light [Chromo] therapy and Sound therapy...both vibrational energy methods. I have, and use, a Crystal Light Table that combines crystal, magnetic, light, and sound therapy, all in one amazing healing experience. I also use fine hand cut crystals, both with the Crystal Light Table and directly in my hands, to focus the energy that courses through my system, to treat specific issues and areas that are generally pain related.

Clients come to see us with a range of issues. Many arrive at our doors knowing that they must be there, but do not exactly know why. Some come to see us if they are in pain or have chronic pain issues. Many have deep seated traumatic experiences that occurred early in life and are embedded, suppressed, or buried in the subconscious. It is truly shocking to read and hear their stories and what happened to them. One of the most interesting areas of my work is working with someone, and whilst "body scanning", I sense issues in their energy fields and see images that relate to incidents that occurred in their past lives. Body scanning is a method where I move my hands over the body, in the aura, without touching the Client.

One Client came to us with a range of issues including arthritis/joint pain and swelling, asthma, cancer, issues with blood pressure, sinus problems, stress and weight issues. Three weeks before we met, she had received stem cell regeneration work for her right knee for what was described by the Orthopedic doctor as "a worn-out knee with Osteoarthritis." For 9 years she had been a candidate for knee replacement, but she explained that she "did not want metals in her legs." Her knees were compromised to the extent that the Doctor said that her knees would never be 100% better and gave her a prognosis in the range of 45 - 75% for improvement. Our Client was happy to take that improvement, as anything was better than they were. With Osteoarthritis of the knees, not only did her knees hurt, but the backs of the knees swelled with fluid (much like a blister); they are called Baker's Cysts. She had to have the right one drained several times. When she started working with us, she had to hold on to the rail by the eleven steps that lead up to the front door of the center…the pain in her left knee was so bad.

We would treat her using several different techniques. I would use the Crystal Light Table, that combines magnetic therapy, light or Chromotherapy, sound therapy and Crystal therapy to treat her. The large fine hand cut crystal was programed with her intention for healing. Chakra colored light was beamed through the crystal located behind her head into her aura and chakras. It is a very enveloping or cocooning feeling as the lights do their work. I would start the session with a guided meditation so that she would relax; releasing her negative thoughts and fears, releasing all things that did not serve her highest good. As the chakra-colored light, flooded through the crystal, from red (the root chakra) to violet (the crown chakra) I would play the corresponding chakra crystal singing bowls. It is a truly amazing experience.

I would also use focused approaches, using either just my hands, or a special hand-cut crystal held to focus the energy at specific areas to remove or disperse the pain. I would hover my hands over her knees, and she could feel heat coming from my hands. As part of the treatment I asked the Client to let go of all negative thoughts and feelings, and these would be replaced by the desire that her knees would heal, and I would instill positive affirmations that she was pain free.

She would always judge how her knees felt after working with me by not having to hold the handrails going down the stairs after our sessions. After several sessions, she did not have the kind of swelling behind her knees that she previously had. She felt good and could walk 4 - 5 miles, when previously she could not even walk one block without being in pain, even after the stem cell regeneration work.

She worked with us each week for approximately six months. During that time, her business increased dramatically. We believe that once you change your energy, the way you present yourself to the world and others changes. You become more attractive and approachable as you cast off your negative feelings.

We also worked on her using colorpuncture (acupuncture without needles, or like acupuncture but using crystals and light beams). We used these to deal with her allergy and sinus issues, an ongoing Thyroid issue, sleep issues, and things that stemmed from conflict in her earlier life. Every time she left us, she reported that she "felt refreshed beyond belief and took on her week to a much more productive and happy level".

This is all well and good, and a fabulous success story. Does it hold up to scrutiny? Well yes, our Client's Doctor took X-rays of her knees. He was very surprised! When reviewing the results, for the first time in the nine years that they have been monitoring her knees, her cartilage had not deteriorated any more. A cynic could say that the improvement was due to the platelet-rich plasma treatments, but this was only performed on one knee and she could only walk one block without being in pain before our work. Could it be a combination of the Integrative Benefits of Alternative therapy?

This is one of many clients and case studies. It may seem to be simply pain relief, but it was so much more. Over time, you can see her increasing business success and "feeling refreshed beyond belief." Some involve "seeing" through intuition the deep trauma that has affected their lives, the negative energetic baggage being carried around, and helping them release it. For others, I see/sense illness that is about to occur. I am not claiming to be a medical intuitive, but to sense that someone has an issue with their reproductive organs a few days before she is told that she had to have hysterectomy, is revealing.

Some clients are complicated, others simpler…like helping an athlete run again after damaging her knee.

Many other cases and Clients' experiences could be presented. This is the power of Light and Sound Therapy and the Use of Crystals.

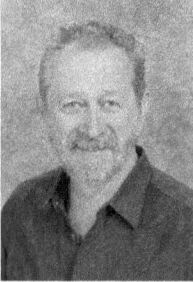

Simon holds a PhD in Geophysics, specifically [micro-]seismology, he is not some woo-woo person expounding New Age beliefs; he blends the scientific with the spiritual. He has worked in industry applying geophysical methods globally since 1980. He predominantly used seismic exploration methods, a method that uses sound waves to investigate the sub-surface to locate oil and gas reserves. He now uses sound and light as therapeutic methodologies to help his Clients.

Simon started his exploration of the energetic arts in 2011 although he realized his abilities at an early age. Simon is an energy healer and one of the Founders of the Iaso Wellness Center. The mission of the center is to facilitate life changing transformations and reboot the core coding of their energetic imprint through uniquely integrated approaches to energy and vibrational therapeutic methods.

Simon is trained in multiple energy healing modalities. He is a Certified Crystal Light Table Practitioner, a Master Atlantean Healer and a certified Master Angelic Reiki practitioner. Simon uses the Crystal Light Table which uses Sound, Light [chromo], Magnetic and Crystal therapies to treat those with anxiety, stress and chronic issues such as pain. The application of sound therapy is a continuation of his work using sound waves; initially in exploration and now as a therapeutic methodology.

www.IasoWellnessCenter.com

Chapter 11
Truly a Miracle
by Susan Maddux

"You can't go back and change the beginning, but you can start where you are and change the ending." ~C.S. Lewis

Shay was 3 days old when she became our youngest daughter. She had a seven-year-old sibling. She was truly a gift from God, since we wanted another child, and I was biologically unable. She was very physically advanced, reaching development milestones very early, and walking by the time she was nine months old. Additionally, she was defiant, and very impulsive prior to the traditional "Terrible Twos." In other words, she was a delightful, energetic, precocious handful.

She would climb on anything she could climb on; tables, chairs, and escaping any means of containment, such as a playpen, highchair or car seat. She would put herself in danger, and her lack of impulse control would frighten us. Recommendations from her Pediatrician, and Preschool teachers, all leaned towards medications for ADHD. I was seriously opposed to the medication suggestions and chose to go holistic in my approach.

I obtained mixtures of tinctures, potions and pills from a natural healing store, addressing sleep patterns, travel sickness, and especially her level of activity, hoping to detox anything that could be the source of her hyperactivity.

Nothing seemed to help.

Shay was progressing through her classes in school, academically showing no signs of learning disability. However, her teachers reported squabbles with classmates and an inability to capture and hold her attention or sit still.

Ultimately, we surrendered to a pediatric evaluation from an ADHD specialist. After what seemed to be a thorough evaluation, a diagnosis of ADHD was confirmed, and medications were prescribed. The first prescription depressed both Shay and her appetite. She almost appeared like a zombie, and she wouldn't eat. On to plan B…medications. The results were slightly better, but still unacceptable. We allowed this to go on for years, trying different medications, and adjusting dosages. We continued on this path since her behavior incidents decreased, her grades maintained or increased, and she seemed okay.

"Okay" is the critical word here. Shay was not thriving, and neither were we, as parents.

As class sizes started to increase around third grade my concern heightened because I actually noticed some academic decline. Three months in a private school only accelerated her decline, so we returned to the public-school system.

Attention-seeking and defiant behavior issues required us to seek counselling, repeatedly, and all of us, especially Shay, were becoming very frustrated. Even though the doctors were satisfied, Shay, my husband, and myself were very dissatisfied and frustrated, but we didn't know what else to do. Shay was beginning middle school, and starting puberty, which was not a fun time emotionally and physically for Shay. I was introduced to essential oils the year prior, but avoided them, since we had no success using other holistic means. We decided to try the essential oils after I read some revealing information on Focus Blend. Shay was able to sample some essential oils that smelled good to her, and my friend made a special blend for her with Vetiver and Lavender. I must admit this blend smelled good to me, too. I have learned that your body will tell you what it needs the most by the scent you like. Shay was able to use this essential oil blend in school. After the third day of using the essential oil blend, Shay told me that it helped her to listen to the teacher, and it made her feel calmer. I got her essential oil necklaces and bracelets to wear during school because she was not allowed to use the essential oils during class time. I would apply essential oils in the morning along her spine and the bottom of her feet to support her immune system and ADHD. Shay learned to roll them on her wrists, neck and diffuser necklace while at school. Although she still struggled through seventh grade, we saw a huge improvement with her physical appearance, and emotional state. Eventually she was able to stop her ADHD medicine and only use essential oils and Omega and Vitamin Complex supplements. Shay will tell you that she doesn't need anything but will ask for oils when she knows she needs them. The essential oils have improved Shay's mood dramatically. So much so, that her relationships with her peers have strengthened. She makes friends easily, and now has normal relationships for her age.

I have learned so much about essential oils, through other users and education classes. I have the top ten essential oils on hand as part of our medicine cabinet, and I love teaching my husband, Shay and others how to use only certified pure, therapeutic grade, quality essential oils. I can't imagine where we would be today managing Shay's ADHD, impulse control, and defiant disorder, if we had not decided to try oils.

Through being an advocate for my daughter, proper testing was finally done, which prompted a diagnosis as High Functioning Autism. You have a choice to control what you put on or use in your body. Listen to your gut instinct. I'm so happy that I made the choice of using essential oils for my families emotional and physical needs. I have not only helped Shay with her ADHD, but I was also able to help ease my husband's back pain. I use essential oils daily to support our digestive issues, mood, sleep and many other ailments that come our way. I have helped a friend that suffered from severe aching feet after a long day of work with Deep Blue Rub, and many other friends, family, and people I have met on this journey with me to improve their health and emotional wellness.

Essential oil use is not new; they have been used since biblical times. Be cautious of essential oils on the market today. Most of them are adulterated with harmful additives and fillers.

Certified Pure Therapeutic Grade Quality essential oils can be used aromatically, topically on the skin where needed, and internally. I have used essential oils in all three ways, but one of my favorites is using them aromatically in an essential oil diffuser, because you will still benefit from getting the therapeutic properties of the oils in your body. Science is truly amazing!

My extensive experience with essential oils inspires me to share with anyone who suffers from ailments that persist with traditional medicine.

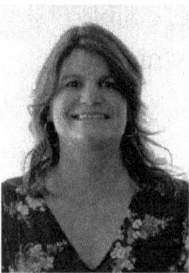

Susan Maddux is an author, special needs child advocate, essential oil wellness advocate, certified medical assistant and certified in Aroma Touch Massage with essential oils.

After struggling with infertility, and having to go through IVF, she gave birth to her first daughter in 1996, then was blessed with the private adoption of a newborn baby girl, Shay, in June 2004.

Shay reached milestones very early, is very smart and beautiful. It wasn't until she started school and showed signs of attention problems that she was diagnosed with Attention Deficit Hyperactivity Disorder (ADHD). After years of trying different remedies, mom discovered the answer to her prayers…certified pure therapeutic grade essential oils.

Susan was introduced to essential oils in 2016 and knew she had to be a part of the essential oil company as a wellness advocate.

It is her mission to share the power of essential oils for pain, stress, digestive issues, sleep and specifically for children, ADHD symptoms.

Her biggest passion now is continuing to learn everything she can about essential oils, so that she can teach you to be empowered using mother nature's most precious gift of plants, trees and flowers that provide us with natural alternative medicine, essential oils.

www.SusanGMaddux.com

Chapter 12

How Creativity Heals: Two Modalities Towards Healing

by Christi Corradi

Our imagination is the most important faculty we possess. It can be our greatest resource or our most formidable adversary. It is through our imagination that we discern possibilities and options... imagination is the deepest voice of the soul and can be heard clearly only through cultivation and careful attention. A relationship with our imagination is a relationship with our deepest self. – Pat B. Allen

As a young adult, I moved alone with my cat from the wholesome Pacific Northwest to plastic lightning-paced Southern California, expecting to find gold and the American dream. Instead, I was faced with the reality of a room in someone's home who quickly evicted me, for no known reason. I started a job selling advertising, which ended abruptly when I was fired for, no known reason. After finding another place to stay, my only companion, my beautiful cat, was eaten by coyotes. My next position was with a construction crew where both my employer and I were seriously injured, and he found me at fault for the accident. I was terminated, and I was so injured that I was unable to work.

I saw a chiropractor who recognized that, in addition to my physical injuries, I was in a terrible state of victimhood. She referred me to Dr. Peggy Bassett, a spiritual teacher who ministered to a very large congregation.

While my young life was crumbling, it was a blessing to find a teacher and mentor, Dr. Peggy, who opened her arms, and my heart, and she saved my life. Dr. Peggy's statement was: "We are a place for you to find your own Divinity, whatever that may be."

Under Dr. Peggy's guidance, I began to explore the Universal Laws, the laws that are invisible, and hidden from common understanding, that actually govern our outcomes.

Gradually, I reversed the negative spiral of my life. I went to graduate school, met my husband, and began teaching these principles in various venues where I inspired young people with these ideas.

With gratitude for their permission, I share my clients' stories anonymously.

Melinda, suffering from clinical depression, entered my youth empowerment program, where she learned a deeper way of navigating life. She went off to college, then married and had a baby. Although improved, she was still coping with clinical depression.

She reached out to me after almost 10 years, with a desire for my guidance. I was creating my system, Mastering the Art of Life, which begins with The Creative Way, a full year of material and training, and I now had a method that I could use to really help her. We looked at the principles I was teaching and applied them to her desires and discontents. Melinda expressed two longings. One; to have a second child. Her first son was seven and she hadn't been able to have another baby. Two; to work at a nursery, teaching gardening, possibly to kids.

In creating a vision, I asked Melinda to imagine her longings. When she thought about getting pregnant, she found it hard to imagine, since she had lost a couple of pregnancies. However, she was able to imagine the gardening job. And she did get a gardening job, began teaching, and used Creative Thinking to help others, and herself. It built her confidence, her belief in herself, and her intuition - and that created a miracle!

Melinda got pregnant again, but unfortunately, once again she lost the baby. The doctor confirmed it and gave her medicine to clear things out. When she recalled the experience to me, she said, "Christi, for the first time I believed in myself instead of the doctor, and people outside of me." She went back the next day, without taking the medication, and told the doctor she wasn't going to take it. He did an ultrasound and found there was a second fetus. And that little miracle baby is Owen, often heard in the background of our coaching calls! Learning to trust herself was a powerful tool for Melinda.

It has been a long bumpy road, and the art-making process has been an integral part of the healing journey for Sheila, a curious and very quiet young woman who attended my workshop. She was creative, looking for help, and became a client. As we worked together, she began trusting me and the process, slowly revealing her history.

Sheila had grown up with two older brothers. Their family appeared normal, but for Sheila it was treacherous. Her mother was controlling, placing a high value on appearances. She was unskilled as a mother, not loving, and very needy herself. Sheila's father gave in to everything the mother dictated. With focus on what the outside world would see and think of them, the toxic inside world was hidden. Sheila's oldest brother began molesting her. When she told her parents - the ones meant to keep her safe - they refused to listen, turned away, and shamed her into keeping quiet.

As a result of this very dysfunctional family situation, Sheila, as a young girl, developed multiple personalities to hold the different parts of her fears and pain, and keep her safe. Her diagnosis (Dissociative Identity Disorder) was actually an amazing system to save her life. When she came to work with me, she had been getting support from both psychologists and psychiatrists.

In her interior system was a baby that needed feeding and nurturing; a little boy, the protector; and two younger girls, one holding the picture of all being well; the other, "Andrea," holding the pain. Teenaged "Sylvia" held the normal teenage angst. In my work with Sheila, art was used for the various parts; first to build trust, then to restore experiences missed, and finally to teach things she should have learned. The deepest part was the healing work.

One of the first creative practices Sheila and I developed together was a centering activity. I created templates that she would color for the first five minutes. This process later became the key component of my first three-month program called The Creative Way in 5 Minutes a Day. This process helped center and ground Sheila so we could begin our work.

Andrea, the younger girl who held the memories of pain, was the one we most often worked with. Andrea had a hard time facing many of the everyday things that Sheila had to deal with, such as occasional contact with Sheila's father, or conflict with a verbally abusive bystander when Sheila was walking her dog.

In the studio, we created a safe place for Andrea, a small model of a cozy enclosed bed. To navigate difficult things, Sheila would invite Andrea into this very pleasing refuge. When she completed the difficult tasks or experiences, she would invite Andrea out. This began to stop the trauma. The Andrea part of Sheila was very creative and loved to make art that allowed her to repattern the memories of her childhood.

Another experience Sheila found very helpful was to draw her childhood kitchen. This was often the place of abusive interactions with her mom. Sheila and I role played in this kitchen, the way "it should have been." Sheila got praise for helping out, encouragement to think for herself, and if she was playful, the adults joined in the fun, rather than berating or punishing her.

Sylvia's teenager part held a lot of the desire for the teenage experiences she missed, drawing hairstyles or clothing she liked. Most of all, Sylvia held the anger. Anger toward her brother who molested her; toward her mother who prioritized appearances and denied her abuse, leaving her in danger; toward her father who knew and wouldn't protect her; and anger towards herself that she (though a child) let these things happen.

As Sylvia, she created an anger box. It had a lock on it, and we made an agreement that the anger only came out in the studio. It held bottles of pretend poison, a voodoo doll, and other things that allowed her to express and transfer her anger, in a healthy way, in the safety of the studio.

Over my years as an art therapist, this was both my most challenging and most rewarding experience. I do believe that the addition of art therapy to the mainstream work was a huge catalyst to the success Sheila experiences today. Today, although Sheila still has her separate personalities, she is able to navigate everyday life, care for others, volunteer, join groups, make friends, and deepen her own awareness.

The art became the teacher, the savior, and most of all the comfort. I worked with her as an Art Therapist for over eight years and watched her become an amazing person.

These brief examples just touch on how art can heal. Please note - it is very important to work with a registered art therapist or professional coach, who is trained in the methodologies of both Art Therapy and Creative Thinking skills. It is not just adding art to therapy. If you are looking for, or ready to do this type of work, find the right support. With the right support, this work is powerful.

Teaching what I'd learned from Dr. Peggy, and then many others, I began developing my own program combining my understanding of Universal Law and the power of the image and art process in healing. This became **Mastering The Art of Life**, which uses the principles of art as an understanding of the Laws of life.

The foundation of this is Universal Law expressed through Creative Thinking.

Creative Thinking is thinking not just outside the box, but without a box at all. It is thinking thoughts that you have never thought before. It is learning to change status quo thinking into new thinking. It is learning and using Universal Law to create lasting and rewarding results.

I have taken my understanding of using the image and the art process into my coaching in two ways. One, by using image and the art process; and two, through the teaching of Creative Thinking.

Using the creative process brings the subconscious to the surface to be healed. Healing is transforming limiting conditions into new ways of being.

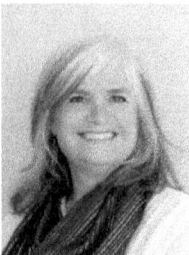

Christi is the creator of Mastering The Art Of Life, a year-long life-transforming program, Tangible Tools 4Success, and the author of "The Creative Way in Five Minutes a Day", a vision-driven program to awaken creative thinking with a daily practice. With more than three decades in the personal growth field, Christi is certified as a Transformational Life

Coach and Life Mastery Consultant. She's also a professional artist and Registered Art Therapist who works with groups and individuals using art, crafts and childlike play to uncover and heal hidden (subconscious) beliefs.

Christi LOVES leading her clients in discovering and expressing their own personal inner Masterpiece, through her program Mastering the Art of Life - bringing out the unique gift each one of us has - and sharing it with the world She teaches how to harness Universal Laws to live a fuller, freer, more expanded life. She uses proven strategies that create results through stopping self-doubt and fear while developing personal faith, self-love, and confidence that will carry us toward bigger dreams and a more expansive business or personal life.

Christi is a paradigm-busting dynamo! She infuses everything she does with FUN! As a speaker, Christi inspires her audiences with steps toward living the best version of their lives - living their lives as a masterpiece. Although Christi lives in Santa Rosa, Ca with her family, she has spoken all around the United States and Canada. Christi is a master at guiding others in transforming their lives in amazing ways.**www.MasteringTheArtOfLife.com**

Chapter 13
An Empowered Childbirth
by Kari Joly' Estill

"When you change the way you view birth, the
way you birth will change." Marie Mongan

Peeing on a stick can be the most—and least—glorious moment in a
woman's life. It had been over 14 years since I had last given birth,
and this would be my third child. The test stick showed the results
before I was even done! The instructions said to allow two whole
minutes to show the results. That's how pregnant I was.

I didn't believe I could get pregnant, much less give birth, without
intervention. My water broke early during my first pregnancy.
Inducing labor was recommended when my contractions didn't start
right away. I held off for hours, wanting a purely natural birth. The
doctors eventually convinced me that I was risking the life of my
baby girl by letting my body follow its own lead. Against my natural
instincts, I let them induce me to save her. A year and a half later, I
was nearly full term with my second baby girl, and according to
traditional calculations, she was a week late. I knew that wasn't
accurate because of some extenuating circumstances. I talked to the
doctors about it, but they just dismissed the information as irrelevant.
I had my second baby at least a week earlier than I thought was her
correct time for mainly two reasons: 1. My mom had stayed with us
for a week and was leaving the next day, and 2. After the induction
of my first baby, I wasn't confident that my body would do what it
was supposed to. Sometime between those births and this positive
test result, I had been injured and thought pregnancy was unlikely.

I contacted Claudette Coughenour, a midwife who had delivered
babies for three of my friends. She came to my home, drank my

offered tea, and we chit-chatted about anything and everything. I asked her questions that I had on my mind, and she used those questions to guide the conversation. I felt assured and validated when she validated the concerns that I had not mentioned yet. I was pleased with her cozy, homey manner. She offered me a manual, of sorts, that had plentiful instructions, preparation tips, diet tips, and mindset helps. I was eager to read it and found the material helpful. She also lent me educational books and videos that empowered me against any angst I was feeling throughout my pregnancy. I loved my prenatal appointments in her home, it was warm, cozy, and peaceful. She had a second midwife, Laura Nichols, who would be an aid during the birth. It was nice to be able to get to know both of them throughout the pregnancy, and they both had a wealth of knowledge and support to offer. They regularly tested my blood for vitamin and iron levels over time, and recommended supplements, which noticeably kept me healthy and strong for my baby. I was impressed.

My son waited almost two weeks after his due date before coming into the world. After 40 weeks came and went, I started praying against self-doubt and applying essential oils. Four days before the 42-week mark, Claudette came, maintaining her usual calm, assuring manner, and stripped my membranes to kick my body into gear. No change.

Two days after stripping my membranes—and two days before the 42-week mark—Claudette came again in the afternoon. She stripped my membranes one more time and she also inserted a gel with homeopathic black and blue cohosh. She told me to lie on my back for at least an hour. Within ten minutes of getting up, I had my first contraction. Twenty minutes later, I had another contraction. Four minutes later came my third contraction. We called Claudette. She said to give it about an hour and call her again. Approximately two minutes later I had another contraction. After that, all of my contractions were 1.5-2 minutes apart. Not only was my body just fine to birth children without Pitocin, it was ready for hard labor right from the get-go!

I'm not clear on how long it was between calling Claudette the second time and when she actually arrived, but I remember this: When she came in, I asked, "I'm not supposed to push yet, right?" It was exactly when my body started feeling like pushing. Claudette confirmed that it was not time yet, so I just kept breathing and rocking myself through the contractions.

They readied the birthing pool and I got in. I stayed on my knees and laid my head to rest on my folded arms on the foot of my bed, where the pool was. My body was nearly pushing, against my better judgment. Every time I fully exhaled, my body would start pushing automatically. I told Claudette what was going on, and she told me to take shorter breaths. I misunderstood her instructions and ended up restricting my and my baby's oxygen. When Claudette turned on her monitor to check the heartbeat, I could hear how slow it was in comparison to its normal speed in the past. She gave my husband a mask for him to put over my face and turned on the oxygen. As I breathed in the oxygen, I heard my baby's heartbeat speed up. When Claudette confirmed that his heartbeat was indeed back up to normal, I relaxed and literally fell asleep. I experienced what I believe is a type of euphoria for a moment. I'm not sure how long I was out, but it wasn't very long, and when I came to, my body was ready to get this baby out.

Claudette told me when it was okay for me to push. I followed her instructions a few times, and then when I realized I was feeling his crown still inside, I decided I was done with this entire process and that he was coming out with my next push whether he liked it or not! I don't recommend this, since he's the only one of my three babies that tore me, and I'm sure it's my fault. When the next push came and Claudette said it was all right, I went ahead and put everything I had into this one single push. I thought, "All right, baby, it's time!" Later, my mom said she had never experienced anything so beautiful.

As is the way with midwives who know the value of a strong umbilical cord and keeping it connected to the baby for as long as possible, Claudette exclaimed over the beauty of my cord. Before this, I had never thought about it, and didn't realize how different umbilical cords can be, depending on the diet and the health of the mother. My cord was milky white with blue and purple veins spiraling around the outside of it and it was thick—probably at least half an inch thick in diameter. True to her word, she kept my cord connected to my son to continue pumping nutrition and blood cells into his body until it finished.

I held my son immediately after he came into the world, while the cord was still connected. Though this was my third child, it was my first experience holding my baby right away, since in the hospital, they cut the cord almost immediately and they clean the baby before the mother gets to hold them. Getting to hold him right after he came out felt powerful, unearthly, exquisite.

After cutting the cord and cleaning him, we immediately put my son to the breast. I didn't realize until after he and I were enjoying this moment of peace that I never used the music I collected, my essential oils, nor the healing stones I had set out. My candles remained unlit. My preparations for my emotional and mental well-being weren't needed in the moment. However, putting them together and setting them out had contributed to my overall mindset concerning this beautiful birth. I knew through the entire process that, should I need any of them, they were available.

I love all of my children. I'm grateful for each one of them. My son's home birth validated me as a woman, as a mother, and as a person, maybe more than any other experience I've ever had in my life.

Neither of the two hospital births I had ever came close. Throughout this home birth, I kept my calm. From getting down off my bed after my midwife inserted the gel, to when I released my son into the world, I experienced zero freak-out sessions. I know now, that our bodies are powerful enough to stay calm during times of extreme emotional, spiritual, physical, and mental testing. I also believe that the information, the videos, the books, and my midwife's overall mindset and behavior, contributed to my calm. My intuition had told me to surround myself with a certain type of person. I followed that instinct and the results achieved were exactly as planned!

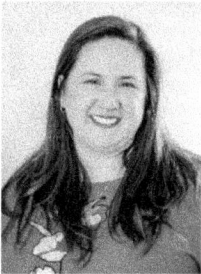

Kari Joly' Estill is a fun-loving entrepreneur with a valiant heart for those who desire to walk in their personal power. Her mission is for each person she touches to value their intrinsic worth and create their own destiny full of love, empowerment, and abundance.

In her free time, she loves to sing, go to the beach, and serve others. She's got a great memory, which earned her the nickname 'walking dictionary' in school. One of her favorite pastimes is sharing her knowledge of holistic health, personal development, and emotional and mental fortitude. Her sparkling personality and earthy presence both lightly entertain and set her clients at ease.

Another favorite pastime of Kari's is helping business owners strengthen their personal relationships, create lasting professional connections, and increase their emotional intelligence with a fun and creative system which she personally uses. Kari created the #TrustKindness movement which is dedicated to empowering the oppressed through education of what true kindness looks like and believing that those brave enough to share it will receive it back tenfold.

www.KariJolyEstill.com.

Chapter 14
A Healers Journey with the Angelic Kingdom and Ancient Egyptian Neteru
by Juliet Carrillo

*"Live the Life of Your Dreams: Be brave enough
to live the life of your dreams according to your
vision and purpose instead of the expectations and
opinions of others."*
— *Roy T. Bennett, The Light in the Heart*

As I gaze out the window in my private flat, overlooking the Nile River in Luxor Egypt, I am again filled with wonder, gratitude and deep appreciation of how my life has changed dramatically over the past several years. It all began the day I decided to step fully into my life and stop hiding my psychic and healing gifts I was born with.

Growing up, I had hidden myself, staying in the background, playing down the messages I received. Each time that I was made fun of a child for being "different or strange," I retreated deeper inside, holding everything within. Yet, one day, this "normal, boring, everyday socially accepted life" that I was sleepwalking through, just wasn't enough anymore. I was drowning and feeling claustrophobic by having denied who I truly am for far too long

I was in my mid 40's, before I decided that I was no longer going to live my life, according to society's expectations. I embraced my uniqueness and stepped out as my true authentic self. I am an intuitive healer, psychic, medium, and full body channel. I am able to walk between the spiritual and our physical worlds simultaneously. I communicate intuitively with spirit, animals and nature.

After 20 years working at a University, I decided to go on a Soul Quest to find my true authentic self. My Spiritual trips led me to sacred, potent, high vibrational energy sites throughout the world. Each of these sacred journeys provided strong healing, transformation, ancient wisdom and deep connection, on a heart and soul level.

I became deeply engaged in finding spiritual teachers. I took courses in Animal Reiki and from there, I found Angelic Reiki. My life changed in the most amazing ways, as I began to live my Soul's purpose as a healer.

During my first Angelic Reiki Healing, I was bathed in the most relaxing beautiful energies that I had ever experienced. I felt a peacefulness come over me and suddenly I felt my core, my Soul, being raised up, held in a loving beautiful embrace. Warm tears ran down my cheeks, as my heart opened wide. I was instantly transformed, as I lay cocooned in this state of grace and heavenly bliss. I was reminded of life on the other side, warm, safe and filled with unconditional love, as Archangel Michael held me in his loving protective arms.

It is my deepest honor to provide Angelic Reiki to people who seek healing. Angelic Reiki is the beautiful healing energy of the Angels channeled directly from the Angelic Kingdom to promote healing within your physical, spiritual, mental and emotional body and assists with balancing your energy and chakras. Every treatment is unique and brings forth the healing that you need at that time.

My clients have shared their transformational feedback on the sessions that I have provided. Here are several below:

A bedridden man with stage 4 throat cancer, who lost his ability to speak, and was eating through a feeding tube, was told he had a ten percent chance survival rate. The man began receiving long distance

Angelic Reiki healing from me. In a few days he could swallow, speak, eat through his mouth and his body ceased to feel like it was on fire from the inside out. Within a week, his body was strong enough for him to walk again. He made great physical progress, gained weight and increased his strength. Within a month he was able to travel to receive treatment from a specialist in another country. This man, a year later, is now cancer free and enjoying life with his family.

A woman who was diagnosed with ovarian cancer, was scheduled for an operation to remove a large painful tumor and receive chemotherapy treatments. She received long distance Angelic Reiki healing from me. Several days before surgery, she had a preoperative scan and checkup. The tumor was gone and did not show up on the scan during her exam. The doctors were perplexed, as they had never seen such a large tumor "disappear" within a month between doctor appointments. The surgery and chemotherapy were cancelled, and the woman is enjoying a healthy, happy Cancer free life.

A woman with depression, insomnia, and painful TMJ from grinding her teeth as she slept, contacted me for an in-person healing. During the appointment she experienced a deep state of relaxation and felt the stress leave her body. Her thoughts quieted in her mind and for the first time in years, she slept through the night and awoke feeling energized, happy, with a lift in her spirit. She's stopped wearing a mouthguard at night, enjoys a solid night's sleep each evening, and has a renewed feeling of positivity and energy.

I provide Angelic Reiki healing sessions in person and by long distance. I teach classes in this beautiful healing modality to those who are called to practice and carry Angelic Reiki forward throughout the world.

I continued studying different healing modalities, raising my vibration and one day, life as I knew it, changed profoundly. I started receiving visions of Ancient Egypt. Whenever I closed my eyes, whether awake or as I relaxed into sleep, an array of Egyptian images appeared. As I slept, I was visited by the strongest, healing energy I had ever experienced. I would hear the roar of the wind, waking me from my sleep. Golden Lionesses in front of temples would appear to me. Goddess Sekhmet had arrived in my life. We share a co-creation of life that is a beautiful balance of healing and deep spiritual alchemy. Together we have traveled to Ancient Egypt, visiting the pyramids, temples and sacred sites that hold timeless healing, potent energy and ancient wisdom.

My first trip to Egypt, was not what I had expected. I knew I would change on some level, by visiting this beautiful, mystical ancient land. What I didn't realize was that it would become my Soul's journey home. This sacred journey would reintroduce me to my homeland of many past lifetimes. The moment I stepped off the plane in Cairo, I connected fully with my authentic self. I had arrived Home. This two-week spiritual trip provided me with deep connection to the sacred sites, where the ancient energies are still very potent and alive. It was beautiful how strongly the Egyptian Gods and Goddesses channeled through me. I stepped back in time and saw the sacred sites and temples, as they existed in their original state over seven thousand years ago. It was during this first visit to Egypt, where I was asked by the Neteru if I would dedicate my life to being in service to them. Once I agreed, I was shown how my life would change. My company, Sacred Soulful Journeys was formed to lead private spiritual trips to Egypt. We visit the ancient pyramids, temples and sacred sites along the Nilotic Meridian, which hold potent timeless healing energy, knowledge and ancient wisdom. We sail the Nile River on our private dahabeya boat, our private, floating temple. You will connect with the Nile's energetic flow, allowing yourself to be gently led on an inner journey to release what no longer serves you and embrace that which you are meant to be. It is my deepest honor to hold space for others during their individual healing and experiences in Egypt.

Egyptian Sekhem healing was channeled directly to me by the Egyptian Goddess Sekhmet through initiation, channeled downloads and integrating ancient wisdom and energies. Egyptian Sekhem is a high vibration healing energy, similar in method to Reiki, though that channels at a much higher frequency. Sekhem is an ancient form of healing taught in the Egyptian Mystery Schools held in the temples of early Egypt. Only select few initiatives were privy to this Spiritual Alchemy. Sekhem healing brings a higher state of consciousness, connecting with one's Soul. Sekhem heals at the emotional, mental, physical and spiritual levels. It quickly transmutes lower level energy which no longer serve you, bringing positive, balanced, loving change to all areas of your life. Sekhem healing provides the recipient with a loving, gentle, calm, grounding healing.

I provide Egyptian Sekhem healing sessions in person and by long distance. I teach classes in Egyptian Sekhem healing for those who feel called to immerse themselves in this ancient spiritual alchemy.

Putting my faith and trust in Divine Source has opened up many exciting beautiful adventures and moments in my life. My life has been transformed seemingly overnight, as I find myself living amongst the Egyptian people in a small rural village in Luxor. I am both elated and humbled by the blessings and magic in my life.

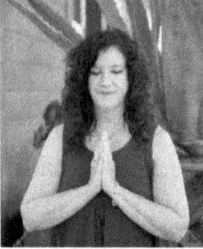

Since early childhood, Juliet Carrillo has connected with the Spirit and Animal worlds through dreams, visions and messages. She is a psychic, medium, intuitive healer and full body channel. Juliet is a gifted healer and provides Angelic Reiki Master, Egyptian Sekhem Healer, Usui Reiki Master, Animal Reiki Master, Metatronia Therapy Practitioner, Angel Therapy Practitioner, Diamond Light Practitioner, Oracle and Angel Card Reader, Animal Communicator and guides private spiritual trips to Egypt.

Juliet has a deep connection to the Angelic Realm. Since her earliest memories, Juliet has heard the voices of Angels, protecting, guiding and assisting her through her life's journey. Juliet has channeled Archangel Michael, since she was a small child. Juliet deepened her natural gift as a healer, through extensive study of select healing modalities. This raised Juliet's vibration to channel Egyptian Goddess Sekhmet. As Juliet expanded her consciousness, Goddess Sekhmet channeled Egyptian Sekhem healing to Juliet, providing her with the activations and downloads of this ancient healing modality.

Juliet lives in Petaluma, Northern CA. Her passion is spiritual journeys connecting to the sacred energies of the Nilotic Meridian. Juliet is available for in person, phone and distant healing, channeled meditations, intuitive guidance, animal reiki, animal communication and private spiritual trips to Egypt.

www.JulietCarrillo.com

Chapter 15

From Toxic to Transformed

by Addie Spahr Kim

*"There are many things we can't control in the
world, but we can control what we put in and on
our bodies, and the choices we make every day
may impact whether we live in a state of toxicity or
a state of optimal health." - Addie Spahr Kim*

I wasn't the kind of sick that keeps you in bed and you know it will
be a few days and then you will feel better. I was tired. I was
struggling with depression and anxiety. My stomach would often
cramp up, but I thought it was just stress. I wasn't overweight, but I
didn't feel good in my clothes. I was starting to believe that feeling
sick and tired was normal. That the haze and discomfort I was
experiencing was just how I was going to always feel. But a voice
inside was telling me it shouldn't be this way.

As a child I remember getting sick a lot. All the way through college
I battled allergies and asthma and seemed to get the flu, strep throat
and other viruses easily throughout my childhood and early
adulthood. I suffered from yeast infections, ovarian cysts as well as
depression and anxiety and waves of skin breakouts. But after the
stomach pain started in my mid-twenties, I knew there was
something potentially serious going on, and that I couldn't keep
living like this. I went to doctors. Had blood tests, stool tests, every
superficial exam without a full body invasion. The doctors could not
pinpoint what was causing the problems and had no advice on how
to get better.

So, I took a different path. I went the herbalists and acupuncturists and other healers. And what I discovered was that I was sick. But not from a virus, and thankfully not a disease. I was sick from years of exposure to environmental toxins. Some probably from my food, others from the water I drank or the air I breathed, possibly the asbestos floating round my high school as they removed during construction, with school still in session. I was also suffering from food sensitivities/allergies that were triggering a host of issues. Oh, and the stomach pain - was partially from a parasite that I likely picked up traveling through Europe and an excessive coffee drinking habit that was causing an acidic overload in my body.

In order to get healthy, I had to detox. I did several types of cleanses, ranging from liquid concoctions to colonics and herbal supplements. I radically overhauled my diet and stopped drinking coffee. I continued to explore a variety of wellness practices into my 30's because I knew I wanted to have children. Given my history of cysts and my age, I was worried that I wouldn't get pregnant easily. I knew that achieving optimal health was key for my future, whether being a mom was in the cards for me or not. I know that if I had not started to educate myself in those earlier years, I would have had a harder time undoing the damage to my body from years of being inflamed and undernourished. Once I changed my habits, my ailments went away, along with my anxiety and depression -- aside from the occasional mood waves that come with the female menstrual cycle, and the hardships we all face as adults. I went from toxic to transformed and was finally feeling the way I had hoped was possible.

But what shifted my long-term health the most was my belief system. I now have the belief that I have the power to not only heal my body, but to nourish and protect it. I've had to rewire my own thinking around my relationship with food and establish a solid foundation of healthy lifestyle practices beyond the kitchen. Making these changes not only took me from a state of toxicity to one of transformed health, but they shifted the purpose of my existence, and I am now committed to helping other people have their own health transformation. After I was able to take control of my own health, I had to do another deep dive after my first son was born and struggled with his own digestion issues. It turns out that he inherited some of my food allergies and then came into the world with even more severe allergies. He spent his first couple years of life inflamed until we got to the bottom of his issues. It was during this time that I became a holistic health coach and did everything possible to heal my son, but also pledged to help others gain control of their own health.

It seems like it should be so simple to take care of ourselves and be thriving from both a physical and mental state of wellness. But for most of us, it's a real struggle. We are over-committed, stressed-out, and often struggling to find our purpose and value our existence and contributions to the world. We are lonely, even when we have a large support network. And when we don't have that, we are lost and often depressed and turn to unhealthy habits to fill voids that can only truly be filled when we arrive at a place of self-love and compassion. This is not an easy task. I get it. It's taken me years to shift my mindset, and I am still working on it all the time. But it is possible for all of us to change, and to make choices that best serve our well-being. It takes commitment and awareness and an open heart and mind.

When it comes to taking care of our bodies, I like to use the analogy that we are like high performance sports cars. We need to add premium fuel (eat mostly plants), get oil changes (do a cleanse or detox program every few months or bi-annually, or when we feel our bodies need it), and rotate the tires (find outlets for creating balance in our lives). To thrive in the world today, we all need to have a solid foundation of whole food nutrition. We need to hydrate, get adequate sleep, find ways to relieve stress, and prioritize meaningful connections to the world around us - with both people and nature. This sounds simple, but in reality, it is harder and more complicated, but it is possible. I am living proof. Had I not been open to other choices, and explored other healing modalities, I would have a much different life than I have today. My two healthy boys may not have ever come into the world. I may not have learned the tools to support my husband and me to manage our busy entrepreneurial lives while also parenting and being a support to family and friends. And I definitely wouldn't have had the confidence to change careers centered around my soul's purpose and my joy in helping others live their best lives.

If you struggle with your health - in any form - consider looking inward and first making the mindset shift to know how powerful you are. You can't control many things in the world. But you can control what you put in your body, how you view yourself, and trust that you have the power to heal and thrive even as the world around us is still toxic and out of balance. The more we realize the toxicity - on an environmental level but also in how energy flows around us and between us - the more we can shift all of it. We can be the change. But it starts inside first. I am so grateful for the gift of empowerment over my own health, and know you have this gift too should you choose to embrace it.

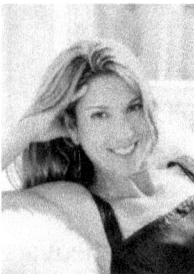

Addie Spahr Kim is holistic wellness, sustainability and network marketing business coach with over 10 years of experience in the wellness and sustainable lifestyle sector. She is a franchise owner with the Juice Plus+ Company and her passion is teaching busy families how to create a foundation of whole food-based nutrition and adopt healthy lifestyle practices that support both people and the planet.

She also coaches busy moms how to build home-based businesses that create residual income and provide the flexibility to work around their family's needs and schedules or add additional revenue streams while earning income at a full-time job. She is a mom of two boys and wife to a busy restaurant owner with businesses in Washington D.C. and San Diego County. She lives in Encinitas, CA and feels happiest by the ocean.

www.AddieSpahrKim.com

Chapter 16

Three Months of Treatment Changed My Life Forever

by June Boertee

"Your life doesn't get better by chance. It gets better by change"

My Dutch parents immigrated to the United States in 1955 with five children ranging from 1-19 years of age. The journey started in the port of Rotterdam and ended two weeks later in New York. I love hearing my eldest sister's vivid memories of the trip. I guess my parents wanted to escape the memories of war and being occupied by Nazi Germany from 1939-1944.

After three years in our new land, with four children, it was quite a shock that my mother was pregnant again with me. I remember how my Dad, during family gatherings, would always make everyone laugh by explaining that I was not planned. The condom broke so my parents were not to be blamed. But I always felt very loved. My older siblings paved the way for me to have an easier time at home than they ever had, softening up my military dad who valued discipline. We later moved from Salt Lake City to California when I was about 5 years old.

At age nine, while living in sunny California, I remember developing frequent episodes of coughing, wheezing, sniffling and sneezing, due to what was inflammation in my respiratory system. My mom bought a vaporizer and put the old-fashioned Vicks in it, trying to relieve me when I was sick, which was quite often. I did have some good days, but most of the time I was suffering. It was such a drag.

When I was eleven years old my parents decided to move back to Holland with four of my siblings. Despite moving away from the Los Angeles air, there was no improvement in my respiratory health. One day my mother decided to bring me to the doctor. I still clearly remember that day and where she took me. The doctor referred me to an immunologist. They drew blood vials from me and determined that I was allergic to dust mites, cats, and pollens. I had no idea which pollens, so I just had to live with the non-specific outcome of the test. There was no medication for me at the time, or anything to give me some relief from my miserable life. My sister had two cats and it was always a nightmare for me to go visit her. In other homes, I would often have problems due to dust mites, and being outside was not a very good idea for me either, because pollens in the air would trigger my nose. At one point, I contracted pneumonia, but luckily, that could be treated with antibiotics. My former boyfriend complained in those days and said that he would wake up in the morning and find tissues between his toes. I did not think it was funny, but I still remember that remark.

Nothing had changed with my health condition in all those years. When I was twenty-five, I gave birth to my first son Beau. Shortly after his birth, we moved to Algeria where my first husband was assigned a job in the diplomatic service. It was my first long-term foreign posting. After living in Algeria for about 1.5 years, I went back to Holland to give birth to my second son Xander. During the last two months of my pregnancy I remember contracting a bad cold and cough that I could not shake off. Right after giving birth, I had to stay in the hospital, having once again contracted Pneumonia. I could not breastfeed my son because of the antibiotics I was taking. My son Xander was quite a cry baby and the poor little guy developed asthma right after birth. I always felt that it was my fault that he did not have a better start in life. I was alone very soon after giving birth to him, because that's how it was in those days. I was weak and could not really take care of my kids, but I had to. My immune system was suppressed, and I was exhausted. According to my doctor, there was only one solution to my problem, and that was a high dosage shot of prednisone. I said yes to that, not knowing what the implications were. I was desperate and did not know.

Full of antibiotics and steroids, I finally felt better after all these years and was very thankful with my new, seemingly magically improved, health. Every few months I needed a new injection. Over time, I had two or three injections and then, as time went by, my doctor in Algeria would no longer give it to me when I felt that I desperately needed it. My prednisone was wearing off, I started feeling crappy again and I needed a new supply. My face became swollen and she explained to me that I could not take those injections the rest of my life and that I needed to look for other treatments. I understood, but I guess I was not aware of what was awaiting me after abruptly stopping with these injections. My doctor did not inform me or was not aware of the consequences.

After prolonged use, prednisone needs to be stopped gradually. My health deteriorated even more, because my depleted adrenals had to suddenly do all the work on their own. The withdrawal symptoms were pretty serious. Luckily, I had someone to help me with my two very young children. Very soon, however, I became sick and had unbearable headaches on some days. They would come and go, and I remember holding my head in anguish. I had no idea what these headaches meant. I lived like that for about two months, and one day I told the father of my children that he had to act quickly, because I was afraid that I might die if we waited any longer. I was so weak that I could not even walk anymore. I was emergency airlifted to Holland. Returning to Holland, it was so good to be back home. I felt that I was maybe not going to die after all. The doctors determined, after an epidural, that I had contracted viral meningitis. A long period of rest was needed to fully recover.

In the years following I was occupied trying to keep my young boys healthy. But now, it was not just me with health issues. Many visits to the emergency room with my youngest son were needed in those days due to him having great difficulties with his breathing during his asthma attacks.

We moved to our second posting, which was the United Arab Emirates, and after a year there, one of our good friends recommended us to visit Dr. Clark in Dubai. This Chiropractor had straightened our friend out after a bad car accident and she was sure that he could maybe help my youngest son, who had taken so many antibiotics, allergy tests and inhalers in his young life. I was so desperate and was willing to try any natural treatment.

We drove two hours to get to this doctor. He treated my son, who was three years old at the time, but who had not yet been able to speak. That same evening, my super active, and probably very frustrated son, started saying words for the first time. I had to go back for a couple more treatments for him, and once during the visits with my son, my doctor noticed that I had respiratory issues also. He told me that he could improve my situation. I told him that I was dealing with it almost all my life and that I had learned to live with it. He was so confident that he could help me.

I could not believe what he was saying, because in more than twenty years no one ever gave me hope. He indicated that he needed to see me for about three months of treatments. In the first month I had to go three times a week, the second month twice a week and then the third month once a week. I had nothing to lose, because he would not use any medication, so I was willing to try it.

After one week I already started to notice an improvement in my health. It was hard to believe that some doctor who was adjusting my neck and pressing on my back could create such an improvement. It was a miracle then, and still is after thirty years. My awful respiratory health from before was history, and this was made possible with hands only.

Later in life I remember telling conventional doctors, and other people, my story and they would all react with the same words: You just grew out of your allergies, this had nothing to do with the treatment you received from your Chiropractor. I know the truth, and that is what is important to me. The successful treatments of my son and I revealed to me the powerful way that holistic therapy can heal.

In my life, I have had two Myofascial release therapists with whom I had the same outcome. I walked in with severe migraines, or months of terrifying pain in my leg after an injury and was relieved to leave after their treatment without pain. I have since become a Certified Holistic Health coach and am studying to become an Aromatherapist, because when I was introduced to the healing properties of certified pure therapeutic essential oils in 2013, I was again in awe of all the natural solutions we have available to support our health.

They give support on a therapeutic and emotional level. I am also a firm believer of "You are what you eat" I find nutrition to be a very important part of a healthy lifestyle.

"Your life doesn't get better by chance. It gets better by change"

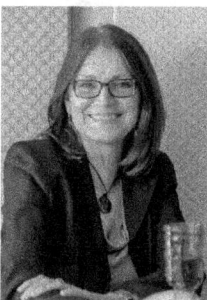

June Boertee is an American/Dutch dual national, having lived, worked, and raised her family in many countries around the world. She has always been interested in the vast potential of plant-based nutrition and natural medicine in improving health and moving beyond treating symptoms. She is currently following her passion and dream of supporting and empowering people on their own unique journeys of discovery of natural healthy solutions. Her diverse background has helped her learn about her own health issues and to translate those experiences into deep empathy in helping people who seek natural solutions to their individual health needs.

June is a Certified Holistic Health Coach, and offers group classes in the USA, Canada, Europe, Australia, New Zealand, or alternatively one-on-one wellness consultations and Aromatouch technique using doTERRA certified therapeutic grade essential oils.

www.JuneBoertee.com

Chapter 17
My Homeopathic Miracle
by Janet Briscoe-Smith

*When you are content to be simply yourself and
don't compare or compete, everybody will respect
you. Lao Tzu*

When I was twenty-eight I had finally had enough. I was standing in
line at World Market, and for the first time in my life, I was
embarrassed to go out in public. I could see the looks of pity on
some peoples' faces, and although they meant well, it was not
appreciated. I just wanted to look like everyone else, and not feel
like I looked diseased.

I got my first pimple when I was in fifth grade. I remember, at the
time, my Mother being much more concerned about it than I was. By
the time I got to sixth grade, my best friend started calling me pizza
face! This, of course, hurt my feelings, but by this time I was so used
to having acne, it was just part of who I was. As the years went by,
my poor Mother tried and tried to help find a cure. Although I was
too young to really care about having acne, she knew that, one day
soon, when I became a self-conscious teenager, I would care very
much. I remember her telling me, "One day soon, you will look in
the mirror and cry and cry!" So, she dragged me to Merle Norman
Cosmetics and bought me the whole cleansing regimen. Cold cream,
and I don't even remember what else. Of course, this didn't do much
at all. By the time I was in junior high school, it was all over my
face, and I don't think there was a single day, in years, that I had a
completely clear face.

I tried Clearasil, and other over the counter acne "Cures", but none
of them did very much. It was obvious that it was caused by

something internal. Interesting, that having bad acne seemed to bother my Mother more than it bothered me! I didn't like having it, but I was so used to it, and nothing seemed to help. So instead of putting my teenage life on hold, and crying about it, I just accepted my fate! Then, one day my Mom took me to a dermatologist. I think, now, that I went through the standard procedure for "teenage acne." The nurse had me sit under a UV light for 10-15 minutes, had liquid nitrogen rolled over my face to dry out the pimples, and then a visit with the doctor. He prescribed me some kind of liquid to roll across my face twice a day and, of course, antibiotics to take orally every day. I remember that they were huge bright pink pills called Erythromycin. The antibiotics worked like a charm! Within a week, my face was absolutely clear, and glowing. Then, of course like any teenager, I thought all was cured, so I quit taking the pills.

I didn't really like taking them, because they gave me bad stomach aches. A pain that felt like I hadn't eaten for days. I would eat and eat, and still the pain didn't go away, so I put two and two together and figured out it was the medication. I'm sure, looking back, the bottle probably said, "take with food to avoid stomach pain" but I was a teenager who wasn't very good at following directions. I then thought I could get by on only using the topical liquid. It worked, just ok, but not nearly as good as the antibiotics. When I went to the dermatologist for regular checkups, he would take one look at me, and get very frustrated, because it was obvious, I wasn't taking the pills on a regular basis. I would take them in spurts. He got quite snippy with me one day and said if I don't take the antibiotics my acne will never go away! So, the years went on, and I took the antibiotics. I would go for months taking them and enjoy a beautiful clear face, and then just get sick and tired of taking them, or tired of constantly refilling my prescription. Then, I would stop for a while. Well, let me tell you….my face sure got back at me for stopping the meds! That damn acne would come back immediately, with a vengeance! Worse that it had ever been! And, each time I would start then stop the antibiotics, it got worse and worse. I was twenty-eight, by this time, and for the first time in my life, it was so bad that I was embarrassed to be seen in public. So back on the antibiotics I went.

I hated the fact that these pills were not a cure, but a band aid that I felt like I had to take forever. I almost felt like I had to be addicted to them so I wouldn't suffer from severe acne. By this time, I started having the very unfortunate side effect of horrific yeast infections in numerous unmentionable areas of my body. They were maddening. I had finally had enough. I had been interested in, and studied about, alternative medicine since my early twenties, and thought, OK, this is it…time to give something else a try.

I decided to check out a Holistic Doctor. She gave me the choice of either acupuncture or homeopathy. For no particular reason, I chose homeopathy. I learned that it is a practice that has been around for hundreds of years, and the basic concept is, "like cures like." Since I am not a licensed Homeopathic Doctor, I'm not even going to try and explain how or why it works. The doctor asked me a series of questions about me and my life. I don't now remember what they were, but I do remember the ones about, "what foods do I crave?" and "what foods do I not like?" The session took about an hour and a half, and she showed me her gigantic book of Homeopathic Remedies, which looked old, and very dignified. She said to come back and see her in a few days. I was very excited, as this was all so new and completely different to me!

Well, a few days later I went to see her, and she told me the remedy she devised for me was, "Silica." As in the mineral that's found in sand! She gave me a small brown envelope, and inside were tiny white, sugar balls. Apparently, the remedy is in liquid and then applied to these sugar balls, then the liquid is evaporated, and the remedy coats the little sugar balls. I was instructed to pour the remedy underneath my tongue and let them dissolve. I also got very strict instructions to avoid coffee, and anything that is flavored with mint. Thankfully, I wasn't a coffee drinker so that wasn't a problem. But I do love mint chocolate!

Well, the first week I screwed up, completely forgetting that toothpaste and mouthwash were mint flavored! Whoops. I had to go back and get another remedy. I also had to go get children's bubblegum flavored toothpaste and mouthwash. After a couple of weeks, I was frustrated that my acne wasn't going away. I called her, and she said to come in for another remedy, as she would adjust the strength. Lo and behold! After a few days, my acne was clearing up, and within a couple of weeks, it was completely gone. I did mess up a couple of times and ate something with mint in it, so I called her for another remedy. She did finally tell me, "I can't keep giving you more free remedies when you mess up…next time I'm going to have to charge you a dollar a remedy." Wow. A dollar??? I understand her frustration with me messing up, but you can't beat only one dollar for a remedy!

That was twenty years ago, and I have never again had acne of any kind. Of course, I get a pimple here and there like normal people, but homeopathy cured my serious acne, like conventional medicine never could. What I do know is Homeopathy changed my life for the better. Compared to conventional medicine, it's ridiculously inexpensive, and cured my almost-lifelong skin affliction, never to return again! I have complete faith in alternative medicine, and I know that if anything else happens where I need to seek a doctor out, Alternative Medicine is the way I'm going to go.

I was first introduced to Alternative Medicine in my early twenties by my future husband's grandfather, who happened to be a very well-respected Chiropractor, back in the sixties. He made quite a good name for himself, even in a day when it was considered quackery.

Another plus I got from alternative medicine, is it sparked me into wanting to become a Health and Wellness Coach. I went to school at the Health Coach Institute where I graduated with a Health and Wellness Coach degree, and a Transformational Coaching Method Master's degree. I am passionate about Alternative Medicine, as I believe it can be a real cure for medical issues, rather than just a band-aid.

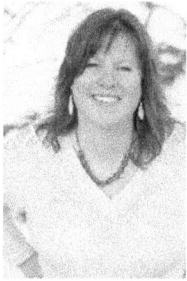

I was born and raised in Sunny Southern California. When I was in my early twenties, my future husband's grandfather introduced me to Holistic Medicine. He was a very successful Chiropractor to the Hollywood elite back in the sixties. Then, Chiropractic Medicine was considered 'Fringe Science', and not taken seriously. He would talk to me about all the interesting alternative remedies he would hear about on talk radio, which fascinated me. Whenever I would go visit, I would read the "Prevention" Magazines that he had laying around. That led me into the idea that food is medicine, and if we take a proactive approach to our health, we could prevent disease.

During this time, I worked at a Medical Laboratory processing all the various "specimens" that would come in. This job added to my interest in taking charge of our own health. I later moved to the redwood forests of Northern California. For many years I worked for a company that made "stents" to help save the lives of people that had heart disease. This helped further my interest in proactive health and wellness. Since my introduction to Prevention Magazine years before, I have been interested in preparing healthy foods. As a result,

I went to a holistic culinary school and became a "Natural Chef." Finally, to further my education into the food is medicine health and wellness field, I went to the Health Coach Institute. I received a Health Coach Certificate, a Life Coach Certificate, and a Transformational Coaching Method Mastery Certificate. I now work for myself, coaching people on how they can take charge of their health and be proactive to help prevent disease.

www.JanetBriscoeSmith.com

Chapter 18
My CRPS Conquer Story
by Kristi Oen

"PAIN is a four-letter word, but so is HOPE."
Kristi Oen

Like many people with CRPS I have spent my life avoiding people and hiding because the reality of living with CRPS is just so cruel. Having conquered my CRPS, I am happily sharing my holistic healing journey with you and wishing you all pain-free days.

Summer in the Chicago Suburbs always meant a family excursion to our local amusement park, Santa's Village. It was something we eagerly anticipated every year. At age 10 in 1986, I was still a little chicken about certain rides and was going to skip the Tarantula. However, my sister and brother teased me into going onto the ride that forever changed my life. Mid-ride the arm broke and my bucket went sailing forward and fell onto the asphalt 8 feet below.

This was the start of the migraines, the neuropathy in my right leg, and a burning, stabbing, paralyzing, indescribable pain that ran throughout my body; settling most intensely in my legs. My parents took me to doctors in that first year; however, they could not find a physical or logical cause for my pain. To my dismay, the doctors thought the pain was not real and that it was just in my mind. Unfortunately, this is something I would hear over and over again throughout my life. At age 11, after a year of extreme pain with no help in sight and no one listening; I thought about committing suicide.

I suffered silently for years, as so many of us do, setting up systems and ways to protect myself from everyday life. When I fractured my ankle in high school, I did not understand why everyone wanted me to go to the doctor. The stabbing pain of the fracture was nothing compared to my everyday pain. Life continued and I managed until I got pregnant in 2006. It was miserable and awful in a new way. After the C-section, my body spiraled out of control and got far worse than I could ever imagine. The pain was more intense now throughout my whole body, my thyroid, adrenals, and other organs started shutting down; nothing in my body seemed to be working properly.

I started the journey to find answers to the questions I have had since childhood. I still found doctors telling me the pain was not real or that I should exercise more. I remember being accused of seeking drugs even though I desperately wanted something instead of opioids. I was seeing up to seven different doctors a week; trying everything for years but only getting worse. The more the doctors tried to help with various treatments, medication or procedures, the more my body would rebel and regress.

I traveled the country to see the best doctors, finally finding one that diagnosed me with CRPS, Complex Regional Pain Syndrome formerly known as RSD, Reflex Sympathetic Dystrophy. He had me watch a video about the disease and I started to cry, I finally found out what I had. The extreme constant pain, the burning sensations, the swelling, and the other odd extreme symptoms were finally validated. I also found out that CRPS often starts with trauma like my childhood accident. It can also spread throughout the body and into organs with additional trauma like my C-section. Things were finally making sense.

Hope turned to terror as I tried the many extreme and very expensive treatments for CRPS including medications, nerve blocks, manipulation under anesthesia, physical therapy, and more. Instead of getting better, I kept getting worse, both physically and mentally. I was even eating organic, fresh, healthy food; and removed toxins from my daily routine to no avail. My body became intensely hypersensitive to clothes, touch, sunlight, temperature, and sound. The last thing the doctors wanted to try was a 7-day ketamine coma. When I refused, the doctors were out of ideas. They suggested I move south, hoping the warmth would help.

So began my journey in Naples, FL. More and more therapies, supplements, and medications failed; hyperbaric oxygen therapy, glutathione IV's, chelation therapy, removing mercury and fixing root canals, and Gerson Therapy to name a few. I became permanently disabled, needing a wheelchair, and mostly lying in bed in a dark, quiet, warm room. The pain was so extreme, and nothing could stop it. I completely understood why CRPS is called the suicide disease. So many people accidentally or purposely overdose to stop the pain.

My mother came to take care of me and saw the defeat in me. One day she said, "Kristi can you do one thing for me?" I resisted slightly and then reluctantly asked what? She said, "I want you to look in the mirror every day and say I am getting healthier." I decided I could do that. As simple as that sounds, it made a difference. I flipped a switch in my mind and took my power back. No longer allowing the thoughts of the suicide disease to stop me from getting better.

I sparked my spiritual connection again and began a daily meditation practice. This helped me attract what I needed for my physical body to heal. I found a lifesaving medical device that I started using while at the same time meditating, thinking positive thoughts, and focusing on spiritual and physical healing. Within 3 weeks I was walking. In 2 months, I was off my $1000 a month of 30 different medications and supplements and off my $1000 a month of various therapies. Month after month, things kept getting better including those insane CRPS symptoms.

I do not live in constant fear anymore. I no longer feel like a prisoner to this burning, suicidal disease that held me captive for 33 years.

I am a CRPS Conqueror and now it is my passion to help others conquer their pain as a personal Chronic Pain Coach. That is why I created P.A.I.N. Help, which stands for Pay Attention I Need Help. I love teaching others how to take their power back and conquer their pain using the holistic program I developed to get me out of my wheelchair and living life again.

It has worked for me and so many others, and we are just getting started. My goal is to change the way we look at pain. Everyone I have worked with has been able to get off their opioids and regain their passion. It is time to honor our bodies and use a holistic approach that supports the body's amazing power to heal.

Remember you are not alone! I understand where you are and where you are going.

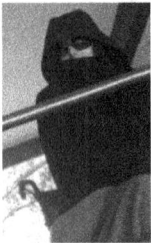

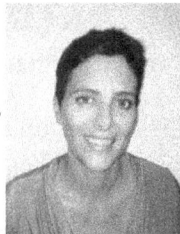

Kristi Oen CRPS Conqueror, is no stranger to pain. Her journey from using a wheelchair and lying in bed all day to living a beautiful life has inspired her to help others achieve happiness through holistic healing and healthy living.

Using the P.A.I.N. Help Program she developed, 100% of her clients have stopped using opioids.

P.A.I.N. Help stands for Pay Attention I Need Help. For 25 years, doctors dismissed Kristi's pain until she was finally diagnosed with an extreme pain condition called CRPS (Complex Regional Pain Syndrome, also known as RSD, Reflex Sympathetic Dystrophy). Unfortunately, the treatments, medications, and procedures made her worse until she created the holistic program that saved her life. As a CRPS Conqueror, she passionately shares her expertise with clients, caregivers, and medical professionals; boldly changing the way pain is perceived.

Kristi now relishes living life to the fullest in Naples, Florida with her amazing son and supportive husband.

She is a Chronic Pain Coach, a Certified Health Coach, a National Board-Certified Chemistry Teacher, a Founding Member and Vice President of the Naples Holistic Chamber of Commerce, an RSDSA Support Group Leader, and a Global Holistic Teacher and Speaker. She has earned numerous honors including Summa Cum Laude, Most Influential Teacher, Makes a Difference Award, and President of the Illinois As

www.PainHelp.KristiOen.com

Chapter 19

You Get to Choose

by Sue Brooke

*"Take the opportunity to learn from your
mistakes: find the cause of your problem and
eliminate it. Don't try to be perfect; just be an
excellent example of being human."*
~*Tony Robbins*

You might not think my story should go in this book. I'm not a healer, I'm not a doctor, nor a holistic practitioner…I'm just a normal girl who grew up in the middle of the cornfields, moved to California, learned a lot about life, a lot about people, and a lot about making CHOICES.

I grew up in a very small town I like to call 'Mayberry', back in the middle of Nebraska. I had a wonderful childhood. We played outside with our friends until the fireflies came out and the locusts started singing. We all left our front doors unlocked just in case the neighbors needed to stop by and borrow some sugar, and we never took the keys out of our cars. At night, we left the windows open to smell the fresh clean air, and occasionally, if the wind was in the right direction, we could smell the manure from the cattle ranch down at the end of the gravel road.

On the weekends, families and neighbors spent time together. We rode our horses through town, played in the streets, and everyone was always out in their front yards interacting with each other. Families stayed together, everyone seemed to always get along, and people took care of one another. As early as I can remember, we learned to always say please and thank you, and we sent everyone birthday cards and holiday cards, and always, always sent thank you cards. It was part of life, and part of who we were.

There wasn't ever anything to stress about, in fact, I'm not sure I even knew what the word 'stress' really meant since no one ever used it! I don't remember getting sick very often, but if you did, you just called the local doctor who would give you a shot of penicillin and send you home.

Everyone worked hard and did what had to be done. I don't remember people complaining about hard work or needing a vacation or being 'stressed out'. It was life…and life was good.

In 1989 I ended up in California. Wow! Talk about a different planet! The first thing I noticed was that most people have garages in the front of their houses, as opposed to the backs of the houses like back home. People drive into their garages, shut the door, and you never see them until they leave for work the next day. I owned an educational after-school center where many parents would drop their kids off at six o'clock in the morning, drive two hours to work in horrible traffic, two hours back at night, and pick up their child after 6:30 p.m. They worked long hours and were so stressed out and exhausted that they just went home, grabbed a fast food dinner, and started all over again the next day.

Moving from a small town in Nebraska to the busy city-life in southern California, I started noticing a commonality in people that had grown up or lived most of their life in the city. This was my first experience with hearing about drugs that people would take for different allergies, stress, and every 'disorder' you could think of. I will never forget a little boy named Joshua; a very smart, over-active child I had in my second-grade class. He was a challenge for sure and had been moved from class to class because of his behavior. His parents, at the request of the school, had him tested. This was my first exposure to the labels of ADD and ADHD. They put him on a drug I had never heard of called Ritalin. I noticed him sitting at his desk like a zombie, rubbing his finger until it was raw. It was almost like part of him was missing. I asked the parents to lower the dosage to the bare minimum, and I developed alternative teaching styles to fit the different students in my class.

It was, and still is, shocking to me how many people are taking pills for something to help them numb the physical and/or mental pain, change behavior, or eliminate stress.

For thirteen years, I was in a marriage that I thought was 'perfect' and was 'living the dream' in beautiful, sunny California. Then one day it all came to a screeching halt...my husband left suddenly, and a few months later I was in a devastating car accident.

While in the hospital, one of my doctors saw me crying and put me on an anti-depressant. I immediately noticed that I was not feeling right. The drug he put me on made me feel lethargic and numb. I stopped taking it and made the choice that I would be the one to make myself happy and never take anything like that ever again!

It was after my divorce and car accident that I started a tutoring business out of my living room and turned it into a successful academic and enrichment learning center with two locations and many employees. After nineteen years, I made the choice to sell my business.

I met a woman at a networking event who was a retired educator, a Christian woman, who stood up and shared her dream of owning a learning center that described mine exactly. I met with her and she offered to buy my business. I was so happy and excited to be able to pass my business on to someone who said that she would continue growing and expanding my legacy.

But once again, life threw me another curve ball...the woman paid a small down payment and I offered to finance the rest. Within a few short months, the business was failing fast. As hard as I tried to get her to let me help her, she refused the help and refused to make any payments. It wasn't long before she went out of business.

Once again, my life took a drastic turn. I had worked so hard for so many years, invested everything I had and everything I was, into the business that I 'birthed' out of my living room. It was my 'baby' that I had raised all by myself, and now it, and my legacy, was gone, along with all the money.

I had invested everything into my business over those nineteen years. The money from the sale was going to fund my new life, my new business, and my future.

There was not enough left from the down payment to hire an attorney, so I found one who would take the case on contingency. Over the next two years I lived on credit cards and worked on starting a new business. People saw me as a smart, successful businesswoman who had her 'shit' together, so to speak, but the truth was well hidden. On the outside I was busy; always smiling, had friends, and a great life. On the inside I was hurting…deeply. I cried myself to sleep many nights. As hard as I tried to build my new life and my new business, the harder it got. Mostly because I was trying so hard to paint the picture of my new 'perfect' life for the outside world to see, that I just kept digging myself into a deeper hole. But I kept it all inside…only a couple close friends and family members knew…actually, they didn't really know how bad it was, and truthfully, I don't think I did either.

Everything I tried to do never really came to fruition. I wasn't making any money. I did a lot of things for free, or the bare minimum. I had lost all confidence in myself and my abilities…I had lost myself.

My credit cards were maxed out and I couldn't make the payments. I applied for food stamps, filed bankruptcy, and for the first time in my life, asked for money so I could eat and pay my bills. This was the ultimate low for me because I always swore that I would never take money from anyone. I was humiliated, sad, and desperately trying to find a way out of the dark place I was in.

After two years of trying to collect money from the sale of my business, I had to make a choice: keep fighting or drop the case. My attorney told me I would probably win but trying to collect the money could take years. I had to make the tough choice to let it go...the lawsuit, the stress, the pain...It was hardest decision I ever had to make.

As I sat in the trailer I was living in, with my new life in front of me, and a clean slate, I once again had a choice to make: Do I keep living in a place of intense grief? Feeling like an imposter? Hiding my pain? Holding myself back from the life I desperately wanted?

Or do I look myself in the mirror and say...

"I AM DONE living this way!"

"I AM a beautiful, happy, capable, STRONG woman!"

"I CAN be whoever I choose to be and to have everything I want in life!"

"I AM the smart, successful, businesswoman who has her 'shit' together!"

Of course, I chose the latter. But how did I get through it all, and get to this place, without reaching for a pill, or something to numb the pain?

- I experience, and share, the effects of the natural drugs, *Dopamine* and *Serotonin*, every single day! I send out love and kindness with thank you cards, gifts, holiday cards, cards of appreciation and love. It is a habit that, if everyone on the planet would do, would truly make the world a better place.

- I choose forgiveness, happiness and kindness to everyone... even those who hurt me. If I ever start feeling down or depressed, I send a card to someone just to make them smile, write a list of everything I'm grateful for, and I thank God, the Universe, whatever you want to call it, for everything in my life.

- I choose to avoid negative energy, so I stay away from negative people, I don't own a television and I don't read the news. I only put positive things into my brain, so I listen to personal development books and I am always learning.

- I choose to be grateful for everything that happens FOR me, not TO me, and I make sure that everyone knows how much I care about them and how grateful I am to have them in my life. Changing my mindset and making all this a part of my daily life has truly made me a better person.

I honestly can't remember the last time I was sick!

Life is a journey...it's an endless series of CHOICES, but guess what? WE get to choose the paths we take. It's OK if we make the wrong choice occasionally because that's how we learn and grow. It's just the universe teaching us a lesson or helping us to become aware of something we may not have seen otherwise. Just don't let the fear, or shame, or guilt, or whatever it is that is holding you back, push you to reach for something to take the pain away.

You are AMAZING! Go out and live your dreams and don't be afraid share your story with others...believe it or not, that can be another form of healing...and you never know whose life you just might change.

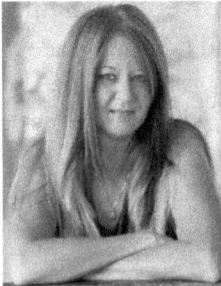

Sue Brooke is a Professional Speaker, Trainer, Coach, Best Selling Author, Business and Marketing Strategist, and Relationship Marketing and Networking Expert.

She brings a plethora of valuable knowledge and resources from 30+ years of working side-by-side with business and marketing influencers, starting and growing businesses, coaching, and training entrepreneurs, business owners, CEOs, and customer service and sales professionals.

She is a serial entrepreneur, having founded successful businesses by mastering the art of building relationships and providing outstanding value to her clients. Sue is passionate about sharing her extensive knowledge, expertise, and marketing resources, and loves finding the best tools and resources to help entrepreneurs and businesses save time, make more money, and help more people!

Sue is available to speak and train on a variety of topics from Motivation and Inspiration, to Business and Marketing including; Relationship Building, Networking Skills, Marketing Strategy, Customer Service, Sales Training, and Leadership.

Send a FREE card to someone who needs it right now by going to: www.CardsFromSue.com, then contact Sue so she can show you a way to do this easily every single day…it will truly change your life…and you will help to make the world a better place.

www.SueBrooke.com

Share your story. Inspire others. Gain credibility.
Be an Author in the Choices Book Series!

Hi! I'm Cherri Gregori-Pedrioli, and I am the creator of the Choices Book Series.

My whole life I watched and continue to watch the Fear that doctors put into us when it comes to our health care. I have witnessed time and time again what I call the Band-Aid fix. It is sad that in many cases we are just a number that is given to us and only allowed a brief time in the doctor's office. They order test, they diagnose and most of the time it is a pill or surgery. How often is the root cause discussed? How often are other Choices given?

Twenty plus years ago I lost my grandmother to a Cancer diagnosis, in all actuality, it was negligence on her doctors' part, ...Cause of death was suffocation. The treatment fried her lungs. They failed to research her medical history - she was not a candidate for the trial because she had emphysema and COPD...What an Over-Site!

3 years ago, my mom received a cancer diagnosis and once again, Fear came into play. The doctors told her that her only chance of 50/50 survival was to remove the tumor. You see once again, negligence on her doctors' part, she had an infection that was overlooked prior to surgery.

Over the last, I don't even know how many years, I have watched Clients, Family, Friends suffer from misdiagnoses, lack of compassion, and just the plain simple they don't know what to do except keep prescribing more and more pills. The number of calls I received begging for help, suicide attempts, sense of loss, depression and anxiety have been off the charts. Common denominator- they were all placed on several types of anti-depressants and anxiety and sleep medications, they go to the doctor for help, they tell them how the pills make them feel and what do they do? They prescribe more pills.

I am on a mission; I have been there in many of these cases and I know firsthand the bad side effects of these drugs. I am here with many others to help educate our communities around Alternative and Holistic Health Care. I know that there is a place for Western Medicine but I also know that people deserve to explore all their Choices. It is your life, don't let Fear make your decisions.

We have so many Choices that not only fight disease, build our immune system, get to the root issues, and more important - bring us back into a natural state balance. When we are in balance, disease has a harder time getting in. I am looking for people who are serious about changing the lives of others, who are serious about delivering a wholeness aspect to health and wellness and are serious about delivering compassionate care for their clients and patients. I am looking for people who are growing their business, looking to help more people, and to change more lives through education, collaboration and connection. Not only do we have the Choices Book Series to share our stories, but we also support and educate our community with Holistic Choices Inc., Holistic Choices Network, and Sonoma Strong Healing Fair.

I would be absolutely thrilled to have you be a part of my passion project, honoring my Grandmother and Mother, in letting everyone know they have Choices that should be explored before making life changing decisions. If my Grandmother and Mother had explored their CHOICES and not allowed the Fear in that doctors put into them, the outcome may have been very different. I am looking forward to hearing your stories and welcome you to share them, along with other powerful experts! Thank you!

Cherri Gregori-Pedrioli

Become an Author the Easy Way...Learn How!
Become a Business Celebrity and a Best-Selling Author!

Compilation books are the fastest and easiest way to become an author and amplify your visibility, impact, income and brand.

To kick-start your life as an author, all you need to do is to write JUST ONE chapter in a book!

You'll position yourself as an expert in your field and have podcasts, magazines and blogs clamoring to feature you.

Sound too simple?

Well, it's just that easy.

Compilation books are a first step to becoming an author quickly when you don't have enough time to write an entire book or find a publisher.

BENEFITS

~Get New Clients, Customers or Patients

~Increase Revenue

~Enhance Credibility

~Land Speaking Engagements

~Creates Opportunities for Media Exposure

The Choices Compilation Book Series is a series of powerful books to inspire people to take charge and make those impactful choices that will transform, enhance and change their lives for the better.

The INTENTION of the Choices Book Series is to:

~Inspire Readers – to learn that they have Choices in their lives.

~Share Powerful Stories – for healing and transformation.

~Enhance Our Authors' Credibility– as experts in their industry.

~Amplify – authors, their businesses and brands through the promotion and marketing of the book.

~Increase Revenue – for the author through sales of the book and leveraging the book to promote new clients and speaking opportunities.

> *"Becoming an author in a compilation book, alongside other inspirational authors and experts, changed my life! Not only was the process transformational for me personally, but it gave me credibility."*
> ~Sue Brooke; Best Selling Author, Speaker, Business & Marketing Strategist

Are YOU ready to become an author?

www.ChoicesBookSeries.com

Resources

For a more complete list of resources visit:
www.ChoicesBookSeries.com/Resources

Suicide Prevention Hotline:
https://suicidepreventionlifeline.org/ 1-800-273-8255

Alcoholics Anonymous (AA): **https://aa.org/**

Narcotics Anonymous (NA): **https://www.na.org/**

Al-Anon: **https://al-anon.org/**

Nar-anon: **https://www.nar-anon.org/**

The Living Matrix – DVD the science of healing

Science Confirms Reconnective Healing- Book

www.ingramcontent.com/pod-product-compliance
Lightning Source LLC
Chambersburg PA
CBHW060905280326
41934CB00007B/1195